SEXUALLY TRANSMITTED DISEASES

Compiled and Edited by

LESLIE NICHOLAS, M.D.

Clinical Professor of Medicine (Dermatology)
Hahnemann Medical College and Hospital
Philadelphia, Pennsylvania

With a Foreword by

HERMAN BEERMAN, M.D., Sc.D. (Med.)

Emeritus Professor of Dermatology
University of Pennsylvania
School of Medicine

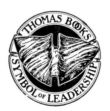

CHARLES C THOMAS · PUBLISHER
Springfield · Illinois · U.S.A.

Published and Distributed Throughout the World by

CHARLES C THOMAS • PUBLISHER

BANNERSTONE HOUSE

301-327 East Lawrence Avenue, Springfield, Illinois, U.S.A.

© 1973, by CHARLES C THOMAS • PUBLISHER

ISBN 0-398-02697-1

Library of Congress Catalog Card Number: 72-88488

With THOMAS BOOKS *careful attention is given to all details of manufacturing and design. It is the Publisher's desire to present books that are satisfactory as to their physical qualities and artistic possibilities and appropriate for their particular use.* THOMAS BOOKS *will be true to those laws of quality that assure a good name and good will.*

Printed in the United States of America

C-1

This Book Is Dedicated
With Affection and Gratitude,
To the Memory of My Father,
Samuel Nicholas, M.D.
(1879-1947)

CONTRIBUTORS

HERMAN BEERMAN, M.D., Sc.D. (Med.)
Emeritus Professor of Dermatology, University of Pennsylvania School of Medicine.

COMMANDER THOMAS E. CARSON, M.C., U.S. NAVY
Chief of Dermatology, Naval Hospital, Oakland, California.

VERNAL G. CAVE, M.D.
Director, Bureau of Venereal Disease Control, New York City Department of Health, New York.

WILLIAM W. DARROW, M.A.
Acting Chief, Behavioral Research Activities Unit, Venereal Disease Branch, Center for Disease Control, Atlanta, Georgia.

W. CHRISTOPHER DUNCAN, M.D.
Assistant Professor of Dermatology, Baylor College of Medicine, Houston, Texas.

DAVID W. JOHNSON, M.D.
Regional Health Director, Health Services and Mental Health Administration, Department of Health, Education, and Welfare, Seattle, Washington.

WILLIAM E. JOSEY, M.D.
Associate Professor of Gynecology and Obstetrics, Emory University School of Medicine, Atlanta, Georgia.

JOHN A. KENNEY, JR., M.D.
Professor and Chairman, Division of Dermatology, Howard University College of Medicine, Washington, D.C.

JOHN M. KNOX, M.D.
Professor and Chairman, Department of Dermatology, Baylor College of Medicine, Houston, Texas.

STEPHEN J. KRAUS, M.D.
Research Immunologist, Venereal Disease Research Unit, Center for Disease Control, Atlanta, Georgia.

ALLAN BERTEL LASSUS, M.D.
Associate Professor of Dermatology and Venereology, Faculty of Medicine, University of Helsinki, Helsinki, Finland.

JAMES B. LUCAS, M.D., M.P.H.
Acting Chief, Venereal Disease Branch, State and Community Services Division, Center for Disease Control, United States Public Health Service, Atlanta, Georgia.

CHARLES J. MCDONALD, M.D.
Associate Professor of Medical Science and Dermatology Program Director, Division of Biological and Medical Sciences, Brown University, Providence, Rhode Island.

RAFAEL MEDINA, M.D.
Director, National Institute of Venereology, Caracas, Venezuela.

KIMMO KALERVO MUSTAKALLIO, M.D.
Professor of Dermatology and Venereology, Faculty of Medicine, University of Helsinki, Helsinki, Finland.

ANDRÉ J. NAHMIAS, M.D., M.A., M.P.H.
Professor of Pediatrics and Chief, Infectious Disease and Immunology Division, and Associate Professor of Preventive Medicine, Emory School of Medicine, Atlanta, Georgia.

ZUHER M. NAIB, M.D.
Professor of Pathology, Associate Professor of Gynecology and Obstetrics, and Director of the Division of Cytology, Emory University School of Medicine, Atlanta, Georgia.

HARRY PARISER, M.D.
Director, Venereal Disease Control, Norfolk City Health Department, Norfolk, Virginia.

ARNOLD L. SCHROETER, M.D.
Consultant, Department of Dermatology, Mayo Clinic and Mayo Foundation, Rochester, Minnesota.

CARL-ERIK SONCK, M.D.
Professor of Dermatology and Venereology, Faculty of Medicine, University of Turku, Turku, Finland.

DENNY L. TUFFANELLI, M.D.
Assistant Clinical Professor, Department of Dermatology, University of California School of Medicine, San Francisco, California.

ODD ANDREAS WAGER, M.D.
Lecturer of Serology and Bacteriology, Municipal Bacteriological Laboratory, Aurora Hospital, Helsinki, Finland.

R. R. WILLCOX, M.D., M.R.C.P.
Consultant Venereologist, St. Mary's Hospital, London, and King Edward VII Hospital, Windsor, Member WHO Expert Panel on Venereal Infections and Treponematoses.

FOREWORD

REVIVAL OF INTEREST in the venereal diseases (chiefly syphilis and gonorrhea) is not surprising in view of the increase in the incidence of these diseases. According to the 1971 Joint Statement of the American Public Health Association, the American Social Health Association and the American Venereal Disease Association, reported cases of infectious syphilis have risen at the alarming rate of 8.1 percent throughout the nation in the fiscal year of 1970. In some of the larger cities the increase has been in excess of 50 percent. Reported cases of gonorrhea have increased 16 percent during the same period, and the situation would appear to be out of control. This incidence of the major venereal diseases is not confined to the United States. It is worldwide. Other venereal diseases, including nongonococcal urethritis and viral diseases of venereal acquisition, also pose a problem of treatment and control. Not only are the medical aspects of all these processes of interest and concern, but many of their effects on the general economy and ecology deserve careful examination. It is fortunate, therefore, that the present volume, under the editorship of Dr. Leslie Nicholas, contains a collection of studies by well recognized authorities on many of today's problems in the venereal diseases. Discussion of the various facets of the gonorrhea problem predominate. There are presentations on the sociological, immunological, diagnostic and therapeutic aspects of syphilis and the treponematoses. Herpes viral diseases are also included. The great military interest in the problem of the venereal diseases is obvious and receives comment from a man intensely involved in its solution. The subject of false-positive results to the serologic tests for syphilis, so important in general medicine, is presented by an eminent student of this puzzling phenomenon.

The editor, associated with me for a long time in venereal disease research, has become one of the world's authorities on the subject. This series of studies by highly regarded workers in the field is a tribute to the editor's judgment and wide knowledge of the venereal diseases.

HERMAN BEERMAN, M.D., Sc.D. (MED.)
Emeritus Professor of Dermatology
University of Pennsylvania
School of Medicine
Philadelphia, Pennsylvania

PREFACE

Pᴿɪᴏʀ ᴛᴏ 1960 most of the textbooks and journals, as well as the majority of the American medical societies concerned with dermatology, referred to this specialty as *Dermatology and Syphilology*. Less frequent in the United States, but by no means unusual in other countries, *Dermatology and Venereology* was the title. In the decade of the sixties, while the terms *syphilology* and *venereology* were slowly slipping into oblivion, the venereal diseases once again dramatically reappeared. In fact one of them, namely gonorrhea, has reached epidemic proportions.

The annual program of the American Academy of Dermatology includes either a special course of instruction or a symposium on the venereal diseases. The recent mounting interest in these illnesses is shown by the marked increase in attendance during the last two years at the symposia of which I was privileged to be the director.

This book is composed of several of the reports read at these meetings. Those presentations which were predominantly photographic were not requested for reproduction here. Instead, several other authorities were invited to write for the volume so as to round out various facets not covered by the speakers at the symposia. There was a definite effort made to give attention to the worldwide aspects of the treponematoses, the newer material about gonorrhea, and adequate space to several of the other sexually transmitted diseases. In fact this expanding interpretation led the Education Committee of the American Academy of Dermatology to modernize the Symposium on Venereal Diseases by renaming it the Symposium on Sexually Transmitted Diseases. No longer may we restrict our thoughts on the subject to the five classical venereal diseases. Yet, not all of these additional diseases are even mentioned. With the changes in modes, travel, dress, contraception, etc., some sociologic factors are included.

In my position as editor, I found considerable overlapping

xi

which I dared not alter. If I omitted such repetition, I would have had to rewrite many of the chapters. Too, no effort was made to unify the style of writing. The papers contributed by men from outside the continental United States may employ phraseology which we consider unusual, but these are always so clear that their messages come across without difficulty.

I am indebted to the persistence of the publisher, Mr. Payne Thomas. My colleagues are to be congratulated on their cooperation. At times, their delays made me feel that this volume would never be completed. However, my patience was rewarded by a fine collection of scholarly papers. To each author, a sincere and hearty *Thank you.*

Leslie Nicholas, M.D.
Philadelphia, Pa.

CONTENTS

SEXUALLY TRANSMITTED DISEASES

CHAPTER 1

THE TREPONEMAL EVOLUTION

R. R. WILLCOX

1. Introduction
2. The first treponemes
3. Commensal and saprophytic treponemes
   3.1 Their extent
   3.2 Close relationship
   3.3 Are they truly commensal?
   3.4 Methods of spread
4. Pathogenic treponemes
   4.1 Treponematoses in Man
       4.1.1 Evolution of pinta
       4.1.2 Evolution of yaws
       4.1.3 Evolution of endemic syphilis
       4.1.4 Emergence of venereal syphilis
       4.1.5 Influence of migrations
       4.1.6 Reversal of disease patterns
   4.2 Treponematoses in animals
       4.2.1 Experimental infections
       4.2.2 Natural infections
           (a) in the rabbit
           (b) in the monkey
   4.3 Relationship of pathogenic treponemes
5. New developments
   5.1 Finding of persistent treponemes
       5.1.1 Reported work
       5.1.2 Controversial aspects
       5.1.3 Implications of findings
       5.1.4 Hopes for a vaccine
6. Summary and Conclusions
7. References

Paper given to St. John's Hospital Dermatological Society Symposium, March 4, 1971.

3

1. INTRODUCTION

THIS PAPER CONCERNS the evolution of the treponematoses, i.e. those diseases caused by pathogenic treponemes. These include *T. pallidum,* the cause of venereal and endemic syphilis; *T. pertenue,* the productive organism of yaws; and *T. carateum,* that of pinta—all of which affect man—and, in addition, *T. cuniculi* which is responsible for a naturally occurring venereal disease amongst rabbits and *T. Fribourg Blanc,* the latest of this group, which is found in some parts of the world amongst monkeys in the wild state.

It was Hudson (1946), drawing on the earlier thoughts of Butler (1936), who developed the all-embracing concept of *treponematosis* for the human treponemal diseases, believing that the four conditions pinta, yaws, endemic and venereal syphilis were all caused by the same organism, their differing clinical features resulting from environmental influences. Others have preferred to use the plural term *treponematoses* regarding the organisms as different but having mutated at some distant point in time from a common ancestor (Hackett 1963); while a third theory, which combines both concepts, suggests that environmental circumstances lead to the natural selection of mutants best suited to transmission under the prevailing conditions (Willcox 1960; 1964).

Yaws is found in the tropical belt around the globe, endemic syphilis usually in desert regions adjacent to the yaws areas, pinta is localized to the Central and South Americas, while venereal syphilis is universal (Guthe & Willcox 1954).

2. THE FIRST TREPONEMES

It is probable that the first treponemes evolved in water and were then picked up by man and carried as commensals before becoming pathogenic and producing the various disease syndromes (Cockburn 1961; Hackett 1963). A close descendant of the primeval organism can be found today as the *T. zuelzerae* which lives symbiotically with *chlorbacteriaceae* in mud (Veldkamp 1960). This organism has been shown to share antigens with its distant relatives, oral saprophytic treponemes (De Bruijn 1961) and those pathogenic to man (Meyer and Hunter 1967).

3. COMMENSAL AND SAPROPHYTIC TREPONEMES

3.1 Their Extent

Nonpathogenic treponemes are widespread throughout the animal kingdom from the *T. cobayae,* present in guinea pigs, to the *T. macrodentium, T. microdentium* and *T. mucosum* encountered in mouth of man and the numerous others (e.g. *T. refringens, T. phagedinis, T. gracilis, T. calligyra, T. minutum,* etc.) found on the human genitalia or in septic conditions of skin and mucous membrane (Willcox and Guthe 1966). Most of these organisms show well marked differences in morphology from pathogenic treponemes.

Others of this group have been domesticated in the laboratory. These include the Reiter, Kroo, Kazan, Nichols apathogenic and other strains of so-called *T. pallidum* cultivable in the test tube. Originally claimed to have been derived from syphilitic lesions, the question has remained whether they are *T. pallidum* which have lost their virulence or are saprophytic treponemes which were picked up at the time of the original, attempted culture. Their growth characteristics and serological properties suggest the latter (Eagle and Germuth 1948; Rose and Morton 1952). The methods of their selection and husbandry may have ensured that they much more closely resemble *T. pallidum* than do the various wild species of saprophytic treponemes (Willcox 1969).

3.2 Close relationship

The close relationship of all of these organisms is indicated by their sharing with *T. pallidum* and the other pathogenic treponemes of a common antigen which can be detected by complement fixation (Wallace, *et al.* 1962; Miller, *et al.* 1966), treponemal immobilization (Guest, *et al.* 1967), immunofluorescence (Meyer and Hunter 1967) and other tests. The presence of this group antigen in all treponemes is the basis of the Reiter protein complement fixation test for syphilis.

3.3 Are They Truly Commensal?

It could reasonably be argued that these so-called commensal organisms have already taken the first steps towards pathogenicity in so far that they do stimulate the host to make some detectable antibodies. Moreover antisera can be prepared against them which will react with them by a number of test procedures (Meyer and Hunter 1967).

That some antibodies are produced under natural conditions has in the past created difficulties in the Fluorescent Treponemal Antibody (FTA) test for syphilis. When first introduced (Deacon, *et al.* 1957) a serum dilution of 1:5 was used, but an undue number of weakly positive reactions were encountered which were considered to be due to the presence of antibodies to oral treponemes. These were minimized by the dilution of the serum, and the more specific but less sensitive FTA-200 test came into being (Deacon, *et al.* 1960). It was later found that the antibodies could be absorbed from the serum before testing by a sonicate of the Reiter treponeme in the so-called FTA-ABS test which, by permitting a return to the original serum dilution, became the most sensitive test for pathogenic treponemal disease so far available (Hunter, *et al.* 1964; Deacon, *et al.* 1966).

3.4 Methods of Spread

Although it might be thought that, apart from fly-borne transmission, the commensal treponemes can only have survived as a result of transfer from a mucous membrane of one human being to that of another by direct contact during kissing and sexual intercourse, from infected traumatic and other skin lesions or by indirect contact through the intermediary of the human hand or an inanimate object, it has been postulated that these organisms are transferred from man to man through the mouth (T. Rosebury, personal communication).

4. PATHOGENIC TREPONEMES

4.1 Treponematoses in Man

It is considered that, once they came to be carried by man, the ancestral treponemes underwent mutations consequent upon slight customary variations in the DNA genetic code, and natural selection ensured the continued line of those variants which were capable of producing lesions best suited to continued transmission in the prevailing environment.

4.1.1 *Evolution of pinta*

It has been postulated that the first treponematosis to emerge was akin to the pinta, or *blue stain disease,* found today amongst the primitive underprivileged Indians in the jungle areas of the Central Americas and the northern parts of the South American continent. Today pinta is most prevalent in Mexico, Venezuela, Colombia, Peru and Ecuador (Medina 1967). This disease, which in many respects is *the odd man out* of the treponematoses, has an initial lesion and subsequent satellite, or more remote skin lesions (pintides) of various colours from pink to brown, blue or black which finally become white or achromic. These, together with hyperkeratosis of the soles or palms, are—apart from the occasional juxta-articular node, whose lesion is common in yaws and is occasionally found in syphilis (Putkonen, *et al.* 1953)—confined to the dermis thus permitting spread by direct skin-to-skin contact amongst primitive people.

It has been suggested that this condition originally arose in the Afro-Asian land mass and was carried to the Americas over the ice-free land bridge across the Bering Strait, between 15,000 and 10,000 B.C. (Hackett 1963). Its present localization in a single global area has been attributed to this region being largely excluded from the mainstream of migration and evolutionary change: its persistence in this area being analogous to that of the unusual finches and other birds and mammals described by Charles Darwin on the Galapagos Isles situated in the same general geographical region. Darwin was to utilize his findings in the formulation of the theory of natural selection (Cockburn 1961) which concept is in fact inherent to the understanding of the evolution of the treponematoses.

4.1.2 *Evolution of yaws*

Pinta became established by the survival of the *fittest* treponemes producing skin lesions more capable of transmission than the nonlesion-producing commensals. It has been considered (Hackett 1963) that, when the humid warm environment developed in Afro-Asia around 10,000 B.C., pinta then evolved into yaws, although some have suggested that the latter was the earlier disease.

The new environment necessitated the selection of mutants producing exuberant skin lesions containing vast numbers of surface treponemes such as are found in the papillomata and other infective manifestations characteristic of framboesia, or yaws (Hackett 1957). Such surface lesions, like those of pinta, remain infective for long periods of time. The absence of clothes with resultant trauma and sweaty skins ensured their rapid spread in primitive communities, and its very contagiousness ensured that it became mainly a disease of childhood.

Through the centuries yaws has remained one of the world's most prevalent infections, but one which, for practical purposes, is confined to the tropics of Cancer and Capricorn. Before the WHO-assisted, mass campaigns with penicillin were mounted on any great scale, it was estimated that 50 million cases existed, half of them in Africa (Guthe and Willcox 1954).

4.1.3 *Evolution of endemic syphilis*

A further evolution occurred in the more arid regions bordering on the yaws area, possibly around 8,000 B.C. (Hackett 1963). The still warm but now dry climate, frequently cold at night, in these areas necessitated the wearing of clothes. As a result of the protection these offered, together with the lesser prevalence of exuberant lesions on the now generally dry skin, the possibilities of skin-to-skin transmission were reduced, and the perpetuation of organisms producing lesions of mucous membranes rather than of skin was favoured as these permitted transmission directly by kissing or indirectly by means of common eating and drinking vessels and perhaps more important by fingers (Guthe and Luger 1957). As infection tended to occur early in life, before puberty, sexual intercourse as a method of spread was not yet generally involved. If, when the children matured, they were exposed to venereal syphilis, they did not contract it since they already had the latent childhood infection.

Endemic syphilis may still be studied today in a number of Middle Eastern countries under the name *bejel* (Hudson 1928; Csonka 1952) or *balash* usually in desert or near desert regions. It is found also in parts of Africa bordering on the Sahara desert in the north (Basset and Boiron 1965) and around the Kalahari desert in the south in Rhodesia—where, under the name *njovera* it was found by the writer in 1949 while making a survey (Willcox 1951)—and adjacent Bechuanaland (Murray, *et al.* 1956). It also exists in present-day Transvaal in the South African Karroo (Du Toit 1969).

Foci were present in Europe in Bosnia, Yugoslavia even after World War II (Grin 1953), although it has since been eradicated. Between the wars it extended over wide areas of the southern U.S.S.R., Turkey and the then Palestine. There are many historical examples, including the *sibbens* of Scotland, the *button scurvy* of Ireland and the *radesyge* of Norway (Lancereux 1868).

4.1.4 *Emergence of venereal syphilis*

Venereal syphilis emerges from endemic syphilis only when primitive customs and unhygienic habits are discarded permitting some young persons to grow up and escape the childhood infection. These persons are now susceptible to *T. pallidum* when they are exposed to it sexually, and syphilis thus evolves into a venereal disease as the only hope of survival of the treponeme (Willcox 1953; 1955). During the period of transition, while some unhygienic habits still persist, both venereal and nonvenereal syphilis may be found together with more older persons being affected by the latter as the prevalence of the childhood infection wanes.

It is probable that endemic syphilis was rampant in Europe in earlier times when its late manifestations, in the absence of any venereal relationship, would have been attributed to *leprosy*. With the improvement of social conditions, and advancement and dissemination of knowledge following the introduction of the printing press, syphilis came to be recognized in Europe as a venereal infection at the end of the fifteenth century. That

Columbus was incriminated for this state of affairs has its modern equivalent in the bad weather being attributed to the astronauts and space travel!

4.1.5 *Influence of migration*

All of the treponematoses have been distributed during Man's mass migrations (Hudson 1965), including pilgrimages to Mecca (Hudson 1963) and the African slave trade (Hudson 1964). The traditional rôle of the seaman and soldier in the spread of all forms of venereal disease including syphilis is well known, and in modern times of no less importance are the migrations of persons in search of work or fleeing from oppression as well as the current *travel explosion* by tourists (Guthe and Willcox 1971).

4.1.6 *Reversal of disease patterns*

If social conditions deteriorate, as in times of war or in a depressed economy, overcrowding results, and venereal syphilis may revert to its nonvenereal form with children once more involved (Murrell and Gray 1947; Fejer 1948; Eisenberg, *et al.* 1949; Rajam and Rangiah 1952; Ress 1954; Taylor 1954). A more recent example (Luger 1969) concerned a family living in a modern so-called luxury flat in Vienna but under overcrowded conditions so that the cost of the television and other sophisticated amenities could be shared with a greater number.

Syphilis also tends to replace yaws when the herd immunity to it has been removed by the mass treatment of yaws (Guthe and Idsøe 1968) or when yaws areas become more urbanized with the population becoming more civilized, with the wearing of clothes, etc., which also lead to a reduction in yaws prevalence (e.g. as happened in Tahiti—Van de Sluis 1969).

4.2 Treponematoses in Animals

4.2.1 *Experimental infections*

Overt lesions can be produced experimentally in primates by *T. pallidum* and *T. pertenue*. *T. carateum* has in the past proved refractory in its establishment in animals, but recently chimpanzees have been successfully inoculated and typical distinctive lesions have resulted (Kuhn 1968; 1970).

Many other animals can be experimentally infected, but their capacity to develop lesions vary. *T. pallidum* of syphilis evokes lesions more readily in the rabbit than in the hamster (Vaisman, *et al.* 1964), *T. pertenue* the reverse (Gastinel, *et al.* 1963). In the rabbit differences have been described in the lesions according to whether the infecting organisms were derived from cases of venereal syphilis or yaws, with those produced by treponemes from endemic syphilis (Turner and Hollander 1957). These differences have been attributed to the amount of mucopolysaccharide produced by each strain (Guthe and Luger 1957). Both organisms produce asymptomatic infections in these animals, and do so as a rule in the rat or mouse. The guinea pig, on the other hand, has been stated as showing no lesions when inoculated with yaws treponemes, seldom showing any with strains from patients with venereal syphilis but as being susceptible to treponemes from cases of endemic syphilis (Paris Hamelin, *et al.* 1968). Only one instance of the successful inoculation of a rabbit with *T. carateum* has been reported (Léon Blanco and Oteiza 1945).

These differences in pattern, although not entirely clear cut, represent perhaps the strongest evidence for the organisms to be regarded as having evolved into separate if still closely related entities. Moreover, differences in the patterns induced in animals have also been noted between treponemes from human cases of endemic syphilis and the Nichols rabbit-adapted strain (Malgras, *et al.* 1969), and likewise a small antigenic difference has been observed between human and rabbit-adapted *T. pallidum* (Miller, *et al.* 1969), although the Nichols strain, which has been propagated in the rabbit since 1910, is still virulent for man as the occasional laboratory accident indicates (Chacko 1966).

4.2.2 *Natural infections*

a. *In the rabbit.* A naturally occurring venereal disease (venereal spirochaetosis; pallidoidosis; cuniculosis) is found amongst wild rabbits. The condition was first described by Ross (1912) and Bayon (1913). Caused by *T. cuniculi*, which morphological-

ly resembles *T. pallidum,* it was for fifty years the only pathogenic treponeme known to affect animals in the wild state. It has
been regarded as having arisen from the same ancestral treponeme as those affecting man but which has run a parallel evolutionary course in the rabbit (Hackett 1963).

Genital lesions are encountered in the infected animals from
which the organism can be recovered. Animals develop positive
serological reactions to tests for syphilis not only to complement
fixation and flocculation procedures, but also to agglutination
(Turner and Hollander 1957), treponemal immobilization
(Smith and Pesetsky 1967) and other tests. Cuniculosis therefore has to be rigidly excluded from laboratory rabbits used for
treponemal research when purchased from outside sources.

Repeated unsuccessful efforts have been made to infect apes
and man with *T. cuniculi,* although some (e.g. Smith and
Pesetsky 1967) have suggested that on present evidence this
should not be assumed to be impossible.

b. *In the monkey.* More recently evidence has been forthcom-
ing about a latent reservoir of treponematosis in the *cyno-
cephalus* monkey. The first suspicion arose when positive TPI
and FTA reactions were found in sera from African monkeys
but not in those from other regions (Fribourg Blanc, *et al.*
1963). Treponemes resembling *T. pallidum* (or *T. pertenue,
T. carateum* or *T. cuniculi*) have since been identified in the
popliteal lymph nodes of seropositive animals by direct immunofluorescence, but no other obvious abnormalities have been
found in the affected animals at autopsy and neither have they
been recovered from lymph nodes from other sites (Fribourg
Blanc, *et al.* 1966).

Whether the organism concerned is *T. pertenue,* as seems possible as the animals were drawn from a yaws area, or some other
treponeme which has followed a separate course in the monkey
as has *T. cuniculi* in the rabbit, is not known. However, it has
lately been shown that it can be passaged to the hamster (Fribourg Blanc 1971), and also to the monkey (Sepetjian, *et al.*
1969), in which lesions are produced resembling those of yaws.
Currently inoculations into humans are being undertaken (Medina 1971).

As it has been shown in respect to *T. pallidum*, organisms which are infective to rabbits can be carried in the blood of monkeys which are both TPI and FTA negative (Wells and Smith 1967), further investigations as to the presence or absence of these organisms in seronegative animals are also required.

That only the popliteal lymph nodes have been involved suggests the organism may well have entered through the legs.

4.3 Relationship of Pathogenic Treponemes

Although some minor distinctions between the pathogenic treponemes have been claimed (Ovchinnikov and Delektorskij 1970; Ovchinnikov, *et al.* 1970), no clear-cut morphological differences have been noted—even under the electron microscope. All, too, may evoke not only reagin antibodies in the host, which are detectable using lipoid material as antigens, but also group antibodies common to the cultivable nonpathogenic treponemes and antibodies which are specific to pathogenic treponemes as a whole, the latter being detectable by immunization and immunofluorescent procedures. No known laboratory test exists, however, which is capable of differentiating the individual treponemal infections (yaws, syphilis or pinta) in a particular patient, although variations in the disease patterns may be noted on animal inoculation which have already been described.

Other differences are noted regarding cross immunity. There is some clinical and epidemiological support to the belief that infection with yaws may exert some protection against syphilis (Beerman 1963; Taneja 1967). In the United Kingdom, for example, a much higher gonorrhoea to syphilis ratio is found amongst patients from yaws areas (Brit. Coop. Clin. Group 1970), although animal experiments to prove this point (McLeod and Magnuson 1951; Gastinel, *et al.* 1963; Vaisman, *et al.* 1964) have been far from conclusive, and syphilis can certainly be passed experimentally to patients with yaws (Findlay and Willcox 1945).

Also it has been shown that persons with pinta rarely contract syphilis or yaws, which has been demonstrated by animal inoculation (Medina 1964), and that patients with syphilis have protection against *T. pertenue,* although they do not have much resistance against *T. carateum* (Medina 1970).

It would appear, therefore, that some differences have emerged between the causative organisms. These are not necessarily irreversible, and the disease patterns of the treponematoses should be regarded as being in a perpetual state of flux.

5. NEW DEVELOPMENTS

5.1 Finding of Persistent Treponemes

5.1.1 *Reported work*

It has been known for many years that virulent treponemes may persist in the lymph nodes of the host (Schaudinn and Hoffmann 1905; Brown and Pearce 1921; Frazier, *et al.* 1952). It has more recently been shown by Collart, *et al.* (1962), and amply confirmed by other workers (Del Carpio 1963; Collart and Durel 1964; Yobs, *et al.* 1964, 1965, 1968; Boncinelli, *et al.* 1966; Rice, *et al.* 1970) that in both man and rabbits with *late* syphilis (including congenital syphilis—Mack, *et al.* 1969) treponemal forms may be found in the lymph nodes and cerebrospinal fluid even after adequate treatment involving on occasion more than 100 million units of penicillin. Such organisms have also been recovered from the aqueous humor (Smith and Israel 1967). Some of the patients concerned have received corticosteroids locally or systemically.

Although such treponemes have been found in association with serious eye disease (e.g. optic atrophy), their presence is usually unaccompanied by an inflammatory response and frequently by an absence of reagin antibody formation, although tests involving treponemal antigens (Treponemal immobilization (TPI) and Fluorescent Treponemal Antibody (FTA) tests) are usually, but not necessarily, reactive.

Although clinical lesions have been activated by means of steroid hormones in a few rabbits shown to be harbouring such treponemes, the organisms themselves are of low virulence, and clinical lesions have been produced in recipient rabbits only in a few instances (Del Carpio 1963; Boncinelli, *et al.* 1966; WHO 1970). Usually they invoke no lesions in test rabbits or monkeys, and even if their presence can be demonstrated microscopically, there is usually no immunological response (Smith and Israel 1967) except that a positive treponemal immobilization or FTA test may be induced after some months (Collart, *et al.* 1962; Boncinelli, *et al.* 1966). That these treponemes have some antigenic capacity is indicated by their capability of being stained by immunoflorescence (Yobs, *et al.* 1967).

5.1.2 *Controversial aspects*

Much controversy has followed the discovery of these treponemal forms (WHO 1970). Some reported cases have undoubtedly been artefacts (Wilkinson 1968; Montenegro, *et al.* 1969), and critical observers (e.g. Turner, *et al.* 1969) have drawn attention to the absence of their true recognition by properly conducted infectivity tests in animals except in a few instances.

Bird (1971) and Dunlop (1971) have both shown that there appears to be little correlation between the findings of treponemal forms in the eye or cerebrospinal fluid with the nature, stage or activity of treponemal disease, to seropositivity to tests for syphilis, to previous treatment or even to their previous presence, for they found them no more easy to find a second time in patients in whom they had been found before. An apparent correlation has, however, been noted between their presence in the spinal fluid and an increased cell count in the fluid (Dunlop 1971) and also in the eye to increased immunoglobulins in the aqueous humor (Goldman 1971).

In many cases the evidence of lues in patients in whom the treponemes have been found has depended on the positivity of the FTA-ABS test (Deacon, *et al.* 1966; Smith 1967; Tuffanelli, *et al.* 1967). Some recent work, however, has thrown some doubts on the complete specificity of this test (Kiraly, *et al.* 1967) particularly in the ability of the sorbent commonly used to completely remove group antibodies which would be present in any antibodies which may arise from oral treponemes (Tringali and Cox 1970). The treponemal forms have, on the other hand, been found in man (Smith and Israel 1967) and in monkeys (Wells and Smith 1967) in whom the FTA-ABS and all other tests have been nonreactive, and moreover, such treponemes may be virulent (Boncinnelli, *et al.* 1966; Wells and Smith 1967).

5.1.3 *Implications of findings*

All are agreed that more controls are required. Golden, *et al.* (1968) found some abnormal forms, but not regarded as *T. pallidum*, in two of 47 specimens of aqueous humor at cateract surgery, and Bird (1971) found them in one of 14 controls, but otherwise there is little information regarding controls.

If the organisms are *T. pallidum*, they are of altered virulence and antigenicity, which would indicate that patients with late treated syphilis can be riddled with treponemes which may not only be harmless to the host but also protected in some way from antibiotics. This would affect markedly previously held concepts concerning both the natural history of the disease and also of immunity of this disease (Willcox 1964a).

Possibly they may reach the eye and cerebrospinal fluid from an intracellular location, such as has recently been demonstrated under the electron microscope in syphilitic lesions (Azar, *et al.* 1970; Ovchinnikov and Delekarskij 1970), or perhaps as L forms (Ovchinnikov and Delarkorskij 1970a), but in any event they have not been killed by the lower antibiotic levels achieved in these fluids as compared with the blood (Goldman, *et al.* 1968).

Alternatively, some of them at least may be dental treponemes which have been transferred to the eye through the blood stream, or in saliva carried by hand to the conjunctiva and thereon internally, and not *T. pallidum* at all, which would imply that existing techniques of recognition by silver staining, dark-field microscopy and immunofluorescence—all involving dead, nonmotile organisms—are not sufficient for them to be discriminated. Important indirectly in this context are the observations that spirochaetes may flourish in patients on immunosuppressive drugs, and according to the findings of Hanson (1970), who made cultures of the mouth, anus, perianal area and genitalia of 19 different mammalian species, they grew spirochaetes of some kind in at least one site in carnivores but not in herbivores.

None of these organisms produced a darkfield lesion for *T. pallidum* on injection into test rabbits.

However, the efficiency of penicillin in curing primary and secondary syphilis and the early stages of endemic syphilis, yaws and pinta is not in doubt. Scores of millions of people have been treated in the WHO-assisted, mass campaigns against the endemic treponematoses. Endemic syphilis has been eradicated from Bosnia and there has been a marked reduction of clinical cases of yaws and pinta in the areas where the mass campaigns have been conducted.

Notwithstanding as many or more people as those treated still live in yaws areas in which mass campaigns have not been conducted and experience has shown in the treated areas that, unless the environmental conditions are vastly and permanently improved and basic medical facilities provided to limit spread from isolated residual cases or from cases imported from outside the area, a recrudescence of the disease after mass treatment to a greater or lesser degree is likely.

Also, owing to the population *explosion,* the hoped for overall, socio-economic improvement has not taken place, and the health facilities *per capita* are in fact decreasing in many of the under-developed countries.

Thus for environmental reasons the endemic treponematoses are likely to plague mankind for a long time to come, as indeed is venereal syphilis.

5.1.4 *Hopes for a vaccine*

Many believe that the best hope for the future for the control of these diseases lies in the discovery of a vaccine.

Before World War I Neisser (1911) considered that immunity against syphilis existed only when *T. pallidum* was present in the internal organs in which situation no chancres could be produced experimentally in the same subject (chancre immunity).

Both humans and animals have an apparent relative immunity against a second syphilitic infection (Magnuson, *et al.* 1956). A similar immunity has been noted in yaws (Medina 1964). When it was shown that experimentally infected rabbits left untreated for three months could not then be reinfected clinically and no virulent treponemes could be detected in such animals (Chesney and Kemp 1964), it was then assumed that a true immunity existed (Magnuson, *et al.* 1949).

Past attempts to produce protective immunity by the injection of killed treponemes have failed (Eagle and Fleishman 1948; Izzat, *et al.* 1970), although indefinite signs of very partial immunity have occasionally been noted (Waring and Fleming 1951). More recently, however, some immunity, as expressed by no lesions or asymptomatic infections arising in a proportion of immunized rabbits on challenge, has been claimed in Poland by Metzger, *et al.* (1969) and by Metzger and Smogor (1969) when the heat-labile component of the injected treponemes was not destroyed and also, following successful experiments in leptospirosis by Hubbert and Miller (1965), by Miller (1970) in Los Angeles using gamma-irradiated *T. pallidum*. In both instances many injections over some weeks were required.

In the American series live organisms were used. It would certainly fit many of the facts if Neisser's original concept was correct, and persons and animals immune to treponemal diseases are only so because they are already carrying a treponemal organism.

The Polish workers admitted it might be argued that their vaccines using organisms presumably killed by antibiotics and not by heat contained viable treponemes and that their observed resistance was a manifestation of infective immunity, although they considered this to be unlikely in view of the controls used.

6. SUMMARY AND CONCLUSIONS

The evolutionary cycle of the treponematoses has been described. It is postulated that the Treponemata originally arose from free-living treponemes in water which were picked up by man as commensal saprophytes. Even at this stage the methods of spreading later adopted by *T. pallidum* were already established.

As a result of mutation and natural selection of the variants best suited for transmission under the environmental conditions pertaining, the various treponematosis then evolved into pinta, through yaws and endemic syphilis, to venereal syphilis which has worldwide distribution today. Changes in social conditions may lead to a regression or alteration of the situation as regards the dominant treponematosis.

Such concepts are not merely of theoretical or historical interest. The observed cross immunity between the treponematoses renders their study potentially profitable in the vaccine field. Indeed, Thatcher (1969) has pointed out that much of the work required to attenuate *T. pallidum* has already been performed naturally with pinta, and therefore a study of *T. carateum* would be useful.

Thus in considerations of the evolutionary cycle of the treponematoses could lie the key to the future elimination of venereal syphilis.

REFERENCES

Azar, H. A., Pham, T. D. and Kurban, A. K.: An electron microscopic study of a syphilitic chancre. *Arch Pathol*, 90:143, 1970.

Basset, A. and Boiron, H.: Etudes des limites du foyer sénégalais de syphilis endémique. *Bull Mem Fac Mixte Med Pharm* (Dakar), 13:108, 1965.

Bayon, H.: A new species of treponema found in the genital sores of rabbits. *Br Med J*, 2:1159, 1913.

Beerman, H.: Research needs in syphilis. *Public Health Rep*, 78:305, 1963.

Bird, A. C.: Paper presented at International Colloquium on Late Treponematoses, Miami Beach, U.S.A., 1971.

Boncinelli, U., Vaccari, R., Pincelli, L. and Lancellotti, M.: Ricerche sulla persistenza del treponema pallikum nelle linfoghiandole di luetici trattati. *G Ital Dermatol*, 107:1, 1966.

Brit. Coop. Clin. Group: *Br J Vener Dis*, 46:477, 1970.

Brown, W. H. and Pearce, L.: Note on the preservation of stock strains of Treponema pallidum and on the demonstration of infection in rabbits. *J Exp Med*, 34:185, 1921.

Butler, C. S.: In: *Syphilis Sive Morbus Humanus*. Lancaster, Science Pr, 1936, p.137.

Chacko, C. W.: Accidental human infection in the laboratory with the Nichols rabbit-adapted virulent strain of Treponema pallidum. *Bull WHO*, 35:809, 1966.

Chesney, A. M. and Kemp, J. E.: Experimental observations on the "cure" of syphilis in the rabbit with arsphenamine. *J Exp Med*, 39:553, 1924.

Cockburn, T. A.: The origin of the treponematoses. *Bull WHO*, 24:221, 1961.

Collart, P. and Durel, P.: Présence et persistance des tréponèmes dans le L.C.—R. au cours de la syphilis, experimentale et humane, après treatment tardif. *Ann Dermatol Syphiligr*, 91:485, 1964.

Collart, P., Borel, L. J. and Durel, P.: Study of the effect of penicillin in late syphilis: persistence of treponema pallidum following treatment. 1. late syphilis—experimental. *Ann Inst Pasteur,* 102:596, 1962.

Collart, P., Borel, L. J. and Durel, P.: Study of the effect of penicillin in late syphilis: persistence of treponema pallidum following treatment. 2. late syphilis—human. *Ann Inst Pasteur,* 102:693, 1962.

Csonka, G. W.: "Bejel": childhood treponematosis. *Med Illust,* 6:401, 1952.

Deacon, W. E., Falcone, V. H. and Harris, A.: A fluorescent test for treponemal antibodies. *Proc Soc Exp Biol Med,* 96:477, 1957.

Deacon, W. E., Freeman, E. M. and Harris, A.: Fluorescent treponemal antibody test. Modification based on quantitation (FTA—200). *Proc Soc Exp Biol Med,* 103:827, 1960.

Deacon, W. E., Lucas, J. B. and Price, E. V.: Fluorescent treponemal antibody-absorption (FTA-ABS) test for syphilis. *JAMA,* 198:624, 1966.

De Bruijn, J. H.: *Antonie v. Leeuwenhoek,* 27:98, 1961.

Del Carpio, C.: *Riv First Sieroter Ital,* 38:166, 1963.

Dunlop, E. M. C.: Paper presented to International Colloquium on Late Treponematoses, Miami Beach, U.S.A., 1971.

Du Toit, J. A.: Endemic syphilis in the Karoó. *S Afr Med J,* 29:355, 1969.

Eagle, H. and Fleishman, R.: The antibody response in rabbits to killed suspensions of pathogenic T. pallidum. *J Exp Med,* 87:369, 1948.

Eagle, H. and Germuth, F. G.: The serologic relationships between five cultured strains of supposed T. Pallidum (Noguchi, Kroó, Nichols, Reiter and Kazan) and two strains of mouth treponemata. *J Immunol,* 60:223, 1948.

Eisenberg, H., Plotke, F. and Baker, A. H.: Asexual syphilis in children. *J Vener Dis Inform,* 30:7, 1949.

Fejer, E.: *Orv Lapja,* 4:616, 1948.

Findlay, G. M. and Willcox, R. R.: A human experiment on the relationship of yaws and syphilis. *Br Med Bull,* 3:197, 1945.

Frazier, C. N., Bensel, A. and Keuper, C. S.: Further observations on duration of spirochetemia in rabbits with asymptomatic syphilis. *J Am Syph,* 36:167, 1952.

Fribourg-Blanc, A.: Paper given at Colloquium on Late Treponematoses, Miami Beach, U.S.A., 1971.

Fribourg-Blanc, A., Niel, G. and Mollaret, H. H.: Note sur quelques aspects immunologiques du cynocéphale africain. *Bull Soc Pathol Exot,* 56:474, 1963.

Fribourg-Blanc, A., Mollaret, H. H. and Niel, G.: Confirmation sérologique et microscopique de la tréponèmose du cynecéphale de Guinée. *Bull Soc Pathol Exot,* 59:54, 1966.

Gastinel, P., Vaisman, A., Hamelin, A. and Dunoyer, F.: Study of a recently isolated strain of treponema pertenue. *Ann Dermatol Syphiligr,* 90: 155, 1963.

Golden, B., Watzke, R. C. and Lindell, S. J.: Treponemal-like organisms in the aqueous of nonsyphilitic patients. *Arch Ophthalmol,* 80:727, 1968.

Goldman, E. E., McLain, J. H. and Smith, J. L.: Penicillins and aqueous humor. *Am J Ophthalmol*, 65:717-721, 1968.

Goldman, J. N.: Paper presented at International Colloquium on Late Treponematoses, Miami Beach, U.S.A., 1971.

Grin, E. J.: In Epidemiology and Control of Endemic Syphilis. *WHO Monogr Ser*, 11:93, 1953.

Guest, W. J., Nevin, T. A., Thomas, M. L. and Adams, J. A.: Immobilization of certain cultured treponemes in sera from syphilitic humans. *J Bacteriol*, 93:1190, 1967.

Guthe, T. and Idsøe, O.: The rise and fall of the treponematoses. II. endemic treponematoses of childhood. *Br J Vener Dis*, 44:35, 1968.

Guthe, T. and Luger, A.: Epidemiological aspects of nonvenereal endemic syphilis. *Dermatologica*, 115:248, 1957.

Guthe, T. and Willcox, R. R.: Treponematoses: a world problem. *WHO Chron*, 8:37, 1954.

Guthe, T. and Willcox, R. R.: The international incidence of venereal disease. *J R Soc Hlth*, 91:122, 1971.

Hackett, C. J.: The transmission of yaws in nature. *J Trop Med Hyg*, 60: 159, 1957.

Hackett, C. J.: On the origin of the human treponematoses (pinta, yaws, endemic syphilis and venereal syphilis). *Bull WHO*, 29:7, 1963.

Hanson, A. W.: Isolation of spirochetes from primates and other mammalian species. *Br J Vener Dis*, 46:303, 1970.

Hubbert, W. T. and Miller, J. N.: Studies on immunity in experimental leptospirosis; the immunogenicity of leptospira ieterolemorrhagiae attenuated by gamma-irradiation. *J Immunol*, 95:759, 1965.

Hudson, E. H.: Treponematosis among Bedouin Arabs of Syrian Desert. *U.S. Navy Med Bull*, 26:817, 1928.

Hudson, E. H.: Treponematosis and pilgrimage. *Am J Med Sci*, 246:645, 1963.

Hudson, E. H.: Treponematosis and African slavery. *Br J Vener Dis*, 40:43, 1964.

Hudson, E. H.: Treponematoses and man's social evolution. *Am Anthropol*, 67:885, 1965.

Izzat, N. N., Dacres, W. G., Knox, J. M. and Wende, R.: Attempts at immunization against syphilis with avirulent treponema pallidum. *Br J Vener Dis*, 46:451, 1970.

Király, K., Jobbágy, A. and Kováts, L.: Group antibodies in fluorescent treponemal antibody (FTA) test. *J Invest Dermatol*, 46:98, 1967.

Kuhn, U. S. G., Varela, G., Chandler, F. W. and Osona, G. G.: Experimental pinta in the chimpanzee. *JAMA*, 206:829, 1968.

Kuhn, U. S. G., Medina, R., Cohen, P. G. and Vegas, M.: Inoculation pinta in chimpanzees. *Br J Vener Dis*, 46:311, 1970.

Lancereux, E.: *A Treatise on Syphilis*. London, New Sydenham Society, 1868.

Leon Blanco, F. and Oteiza, A.: Experimental transmission of pinta, mal del pinto or carate to rabbits. *Science,* 101:309, 1945.

Luger, A.: Paper presented at the 25th General Assembly, International Union against the Venereal Diseases and Treponematoses, Budapest, 1969.

McLeod, C. P. and Magnuson, H. J.: Study of cross immunity between syphilis and yaws in treated rabbits. *J Vener Dis Inform,* 32:305, 1951.

Mack, L. W., Smith, J. L., Walter, E. K., Montenegro, E. N. R. and Nicol, W. G.: Temporal bone treponemes. *Arch Otolaryngol,* 90: 1967.

Magnuson, H. J., Rosenan, B. J. and Clark, J. W.: Duration of acquired immunity in experimental syphilis. *Am J Syph,* 33:297, 1949.

Magnuson, H. J., Thomas, E. W., Olansky, S., Kaplan, B. I., De Mello, L. and Cutler, J. C.: Inoculation syphilis in human volunteers. *Medicine* (Baltimore), 35:33, 1956.

Malgras, J., Baylet, R. and Bergoend, H.: Nouvelle enquête sur la syphilis endémique au sénégal; étude sérologique, isolement d'une souche de tréponème. *Bull Soc Pathol Exot,* 62:1017, 1969.

Medina, R.: WHO Working Document. WHO/VDT/RES/63-64, 1964.

Medina, R.: Pinta *Derm Ibero Latino Amer* (Eng. Ed.), i, 121, 1967.

Medina, R.: Paper presented at the International Colloquium on Late Treponematoses, Miami Beach, U.S.A., 1971.

Metzger, M. and Smogor, W.: Artificial immunization of rabbits against syphilis. I. effect of increasing doses of treponemes given by the intramuscular route. *Br J Vener Dis,* 45:308, 1969.

Metzger, M., Michalska, E., Podwinska, J. and Smogor, W.: Immunogenic properties of the protein component of treponema pallidum. *Br J Vener Dis,* 45:299, 1969.

Meyer, P. E. and Hunter, E. F.: Antigenic relationships of 14 treponemes demonstrated by immunofluorescence. *J Bacteriol,* 93:784, 1967.

Miller, J. N.: Immunity in experimental syphilis. 3. attenuation of virulent treponema pallidum by gamma-irradiation. *J Bacteriol,* 90:297, 1965.

Miller, J. N.: Paper presented to American Social Hygiene Association and Pfizer Laboratories VD Symposium, St. Louis, Missouri, U.S.A., 1970.

Miller, J. N., Bekker, J. H., De Bruijn, J. H. and Onvlee, P. C.: Antigenic structure of treponema pallidum, Nichols strain. II. extraction of a polysaccharide antigen with "strain-specific" serologic activity. *J Bacteriol,* 99:132, 1969.

Miller, J. N., De Bruijn, J. H., Bekker, J. H. and Onvlee, P. C.: The antigenic structure of treponema pallidum, Nichols strain. I. the demonstration, nature and location of specific and shared antigens. *J Immunol,* 96: 450, 1966.

Montenegro, E. N. R., Israel, C. W., Nicol, W. G. and Smith, J. L.: Histopathologic demonstration of spirochetes in the human eye. *Am J Ophthalmol,* 67:335, 1969.

Murray, J. F., Merriweather, A. M., Freedman, M. L. and De Villiers, D. J.:

Endemic syphilis in the Bakwena Reserve of the Bechuanaland Protectorate. *Bull WHO*, 15:975, 1956.

Murrell, M. and Gray, M. S.: Acquired syphilis in children. *Br Med J*, 2: 206, 1947.

Neisser, A.: *Arb Gesundh-Amte* (Berlin), 37:1, 1911.

Ovchinnikov, N. M. and Delekorskij, V. V.: Treponema pertenue under the electron microscope. *Br J Vener Dis*, 46:349-379, 1970.

Ovchinnikov, N. M. and Delekorskij, V. V.: *Bull WHO*, 42:437-444, 1970a.

Ovchinnikov, N. M., Delekorskij, V. V. and Konigsberg, T. C.: L-forms of treponema pallidum (electron microscopic studies). *Vestn Dermatol Venerol*, 44:53-58, 1970.

Paris Hamelin, A., Vaisman, A. and Dunoyer, F.: *Bull WHO*, 38:308, 1968.

Putkonen, T., Teir, H. and Pyorala, K.: Syphilitic juxta-articular nodes. *Br J Vener Dis*, 29:71-77, 1953.

Rajam, R. V. and Rangiah, T. N.: WHO Working Document. WHO/ VDT/79, 1952.

Rees, E.: Acquired syphilis in children; report of six cases. *Br J Vener Dis*, 30:19, 1954.

Rice, N. S. C., Dunlop, E. M. C., Jones, B. R., Hare, M. J., King, A. J., Rodin, P., Mushin, A. and Wilkinson, A. E.: Demonstration of treponeme-like forms in cases of treated and untreated late syphilis and of treated early syphilis. *Br J Vener Dis*, 46:1-9, 1970.

Rose, N. R. and Morton, H. E.: Culturation of treponemes with preservation of characteristic morphology. *Am J Syph*, 36:1, 1952.

Ross, E. H.: An intracellular parasite developing into spirochaetes, found by the jelly method *in vitro* staining in syphilitic lesions and in the circulating blood during the secondary stages of the disease. *Br Med J*, 2:1651, 1912.

Schaudinn, F. and Hoffmann, E.: Vorläufiger Bericht über das Vorkommen von Spirocheten in Syphilitischen Krankheitsprodukten und bei Papillomen. *Arb Gesundh-Amte* (Berlin), 22:527, 1905.

Sepetijian, M., Guerraz, F. T., Salossola, D., Thivolet, J. and Monier, J. C.: Contribution à l'étude du tréponème isolé du singe par A. Fribourg-Blanc. *Bull WHO*, 40:141, 1969.

Smith, J. L.: The false-negative treponema pallidum immobilization test in syphilis. Pseudobiologic false-positive syndrome. *JAMA*, 199:128, 1967.

Smith, J. L. and Israel, C. W.: The presence of spirochetes in late seronegative syphilis. *JAMA*, 199:980, 1967.

Smith, J. L. and Pesetsky, B. R.: The current status of treponema cuniculi. Review of the literature. *Br J Vener Dis*, 43:117, 1967.

Taneja, B. L.: Yaws—incidence and epidemiology (study in Dudhi Tehsil of District Mirzapur, Uttar Pradesh, India). *J Trop Med Hyg*, 70:215, 1967.

Taylor, W. N.: Endemic syphilis in South African coloured community. *S Afr Med J*, 28:176, 1954.

Thatcher, R. W.: The search for a vaccine for syphilis. An epidemiological approach. *Br J Vener Dis,* 45:10-12, 1969.

Tringali, G. R. and Cox, P. M.: Reactivity in the FTA-ABS test of rabbits hyperimmunized with nonpathogenic treponemes. *Br J Vener Dis,* 46: 313, 1970.

Tuffanelli, D. L., Wepper, K. D., Bradford, L. L. and Wood, R. M.: Fluorescent treponemal antibody absorption tests. Studies of false-positive reactions to tests for syphilis. *N Engl J Med,* 276:258, 1967.

Turner, T. B. and Hollander, D. H.: In Biology of the Treponematoses based on studies carried out at the International Treponematosis Laboratory Center of the Johns Hopkins University under the auspices of the World Health Organization. *WHO Monogr Ser,* 35:228, 1957.

Turner, T. B., Hardy, P. H. and Newman, B.: Infectivity test in syphilis. *Br J Vener Dis,* 45:183, 1969.

Vaisman, A., Hamelin, A. and Dunoyer, F.: Étude biologique des tréponèmatoses expérimentales. Isolement et adaption de souches de pian aux animaux de laboratoire. *Proph Sanit Morale,* 36:45, 1964.

Van der Sluis, I.: *The Treponematosis of Tahiti. Its Origin and Evolution. A Study of the Sources.* Amsterdam B.M., Israel, N.V., 1969.

Veldkamp, H.: *Antonie v. Leeuwenhoek.* 26:103, 1960.

Wallace, A. L., Harris, A. and Allen, J. P.: *Reiter treponeme; a review of the literature.* WHO Working Document. WHO/VDT/RES/17, 1962.

Waring, G. W. and Fleming, W. L.: Further attempts to immunize rabbits with killed treponema pallidum. *Am J Syph,* 35:568, 1951.

Wells, J. A. and Smith, J.: Experimental ocular and neurosyphilis in the primate. *Br J Vener Dis,* 43:10, 1967.

WHO: *Treponematoses Research.* Report of a WHO scientific group. WHO Techn. Rep. Ser. No. 455, Geneva, 1970.

Wilkinson, A. E.: Study of late ocular syphilis. Demonstration of treponemes in aqueous humor and cerebrospinal fluid. I. methods of demonstration of treponemes. *Trans Ophthalmol Soc U K,* 88:251, 1969.

Willcox, R. R.: Njovera: Endemic syphilis of Southern Rhodesia; comparison with Bejel. *Lancet,* 1:558, 1951.

Willcox, R. R.: Endemic syphilis in Africa; njovera of Southern Rhodesia. *S Afr Med J,* 25:501, 1951.

Willcox, R. R.: Treponematoses. *Glasg Med J,* 34:281, 1953.

Willcox, R. R.: Nonvenereal treponematoses. *J Obstet Gynaecol Br Commonw,* 62:853, 1955.

Willcox, R. R.: Evolutionary cycle of the treponematoses. *Br J Vener Dis,* 26:78, 1960.

Willcox, R. R.: *Textbook of Venereal Diseases and Treponematoses.* London, Heinemann, 1966, p. 130.

Willcox, R. R.: Implications of the reported finding of treponemes of little or no virulence after the treatment of syphilis with penicillin. *Br J Vener Dis,* 40:90, 1964.

Willcox, R. R.: In Simons, R. D. G. Ph. and Marshall, J. (eds.): *Essays on Tropical Dermatology*. Amsterdam, Excerpta Medica, 1969, p. 35.

Willcox, R. R. and Guthe, T.: Treponema pallidum. A bibliographical review of the morphology, culture and survival of T. pallidum and associated organisms. *Bull WHO*, 35 suppl. I, 1966.

Yobs, A. R., Olansky, S., Rockwell, D. H. and Clark, J. W.: Do treponemes survive adequate treatment of late syphilis? *Arch Dermatol*, 91:379, 1965.

Yobs, A. R., Clark, J. W., Mothershed, S. E., Bullard, J. C. and Artley, C. W.: Further observations on the persistence of treponema pallidum after treatment in rabbits and humans. *Br J Vener Dis*, 42:116, 1968.

Yobs, A. R., Rockwell, D. H. and Clark, J. W.: Treponemal survival in humans after penicillin therapy: a preliminary report. *Br J Vener Dis*, 40:248, 1964.

CHAPTER 2

MODERN MANAGEMENT OF SYPHILIS AND GONORRHEA

W. CHRISTOPHER DUNCAN

AND

JOHN M. KNOX

M ODERN MANAGEMENT of syphilis and gonorrhea requires more than simply a basic knowledge of these most common venereal diseases and of new diagnostic and treatment methods which are becoming available. It must be acknowledged that habitual promiscuity is more widespread than formerly, particularly among young people, and the indifference towards pregnancy afforded by the oral contraceptive and the intra-uterine device has carried over to venereal disease. The physician's natural impulse to ignore the possibility of venereal disease in the well-dressed or well-educated must be constantly suppressed.

In view of the fact that 4 out of 5 cases of venereal disease are treated by physicians in private practice it is essential that they *bone-up* for their role as the front line defense against these diseases. Many physicians are not yet aware that the majority of states have passed laws permitting treatment of minors for venereal disease without parental consent. Syphilis and gonorrhea, because of their mode of transmission, have wide social as well as medical implication. Their control requires more than a simple doctor-patient relationship. Nowhere in the world have these diseases been brought under and kept under control. A well de-

---

From the Department of Dermatology and Syphilology, Baylor College of Medicine, Houston, Texas 77025.

veloped strategy involving close cooperation between public health services and medical care facilities, both public and private, is a prerequisite for effective suppression.

SYPHILIS

Introduction

Probably no other disease, communicable or chronic, has been as widely studied as syphilis. Control has always been difficult; eradication, to this point in time, impossible. Syphilis has been viewed more as a character weakness than a communicable disease, and such attitudes have significantly impeded efforts to discover new means for control. Most other communicable diseases have received greater attention.

The organism of syphilis, *Treponema pallidum*, is an anaerobe requiring moisture and tissue for survival. Transmission of syphilis reduced to its simplest term is a lesion to lesion affair except by means of the maternal blood. Congenital syphilis will not be considered here. Unfortunately, the usual means of transmission is attended by pleasure, and furthermore, the transmitting lesion is often painless, inconspicuous or hidden.

Untreated syphilis passes through the following stages: (a) the incubation period of 3 weeks duration (range of 10 to 90 days). During this stage there are no signs or symptoms of infection; (b) the primary stage (chancre) lasting 1 to 5 weeks; (c) the secondary stage appearing 2 to 10 weeks later; (d) the latent, or quiescent stage, lasting 2 to 20 or more years. This is a stage in which there are no clinical signs or symptoms, and the diagnosis is based on the presence of reactive serologic tests and a normal spinal fluid. Latency is divided into two phases—early, within the first two years of infection, and late, or more than two years duration; (e) the late or symptomatic stages (cardiovascular, central nervous system, etc.).

Infectious syphilis includes the primary, secondary and early latent stages. During the stage of early latency there are in the untreated patient periodic relapses to the secondary types of lesions followed by spontaneous healing. This relapsing tendency occurs for the most part during the first two years of infection. Thereafter, in most cases, immunologic changes occur which prevent the appearance of infectious skin lesions but not progression of the organism in other body tissues. The incidence of relapse in untreated syphilis is unknown.

Clinical Manifestations

Primary Syphilis

Primary syphilis is characterized by an initial lesion called a chancre which appears at the site of inoculation from 10 to 90 days after exposure (average 21 days). In most cases the initial lesion is single, but sometimes multiple syphilitic chancres are seen appearing simultaneously or within a few days of each other. The typical, classically described lesion occurs much less frequently than the atypical variants. All too often the chancre is irregular, dirty and somewhat necrotic looking or is not accompanied by adenopathy. If, in addition to an atypical appearance the lesion is located away from the genital region, the physician's index of suspicion drops sharply, and syphilis will not even be considered in the differential diagnosis. An untreated chancre may disappear spontaneously in 4 to 14 weeks. With adequate treatment it should heal within a week. The Venereal Disease Research Laboratory (VDRL) test will be positive in patients with primary syphilis in approximately 75 percent of cases (1).

Secondary Syphilis

In about 25 percent of patients seen initially in the secondary stage there will be no history nor any sign of a primary lesion. This is not to be considered an exclusive feature of syphilis in women. Secondary syphilis begins 6 to 8 weeks or more after the chancre appears, and the chancre not uncommonly is still present when the secondary lesions appear. In secondary syphilis there is invariably a reactive serologic test for syphilis (STS).

Latent Syphilis

By definition, latent syphilis is that stage of syphilis following the secondary stage where there are no clinical signs or symptoms of the disease. *The spinal fluid has been examined and is normal.* A thorough history must be taken to determine duration of infection when possible. Thus, latent syphilis is customarily divided into early latent (usually infectious) and late latent (presumably noninfectious) syphilis. Early latent syphilis is the term applied to an infection of less than two years duration and late latent syphilis comprises those infections of more than two years duration. In the past few years there has been a trend in the United States to define early latency as syphilis of less than one year's duration, for it is during this time that infection is of greatest epidemiological significance. A brief period of latency may also occur during an indeterminant asymptomatic period between primary and secondary stages. Though late latent syphilis is considered noninfectious, transplacental transmission has been reported in infections of greater than two years duration.

Late Syphilis

Late syphilis is the clinically destructive stage of the disease occurring after the latent period. This stage is considered noninfectious. The most important systems involved are the cardiovascular and central nervous systems, although no organ is exempt from possible involvement. It must be remembered that approximately one third of late syphilis patients eventually become nonreactive to the conventional nontreponemal STS (e.g. VDRL) (2); in such patients syphilis can be detected only by the more sensitive and specific treponemal tests, e.g. FTS-ABS. A classification of late syphilis is as follows: (a) late benign syphilis which includes cutaneous, osseous and visceral syphilis; (b) cardiovascular syphilis; (c) asymptomatic neurosyphilis; (d) symptomatic neurosyphilis.

Laboratory Diagnosis

The spirochete is demonstrable by darkfield examination. However, few physicians are able to, or have the facilities available to perform this examination properly. Of primary importance is the acquisition of a small amount of clear serum from a lesion of primary or secondary syphilis and its prompt examination by an experienced individual. At times, secondary infection of the chancre prevents securing an adequate darkfield specimen. Sulfisoxazole, 1.0 gm four times daily, will frequently clean up the lesion without affecting the spirochete and thus make it possible to obtain a more satisfactory darkfield specimen. Dark-field examination provides the only absolute diagnosis of syphilis.

Two basic types of antibodies are produced in response to treponemal invasion: (a) nonspecific antibodies (reagins) and (b) specific antitreponemal antibodies. Among the nontreponemal tests, the VDRL is the most commonly used flocculation test. These tests are the standard for screening purposes and for following the serologic response to treatment. Most laboratories report the result of the highest dilution of a patient's serum that still gives a positive test. Quantitative tests are helpful because they establish a baseline from which change can be measured. A fourfold or greater change in the quantitative VDRL titer is necessary to demonstrate a significant change in the level of reagin type antibody since twofold changes are commonly due to technical factors. Another nontreponemal test in common usage is the Rapid Plasma Reagin (RPR) test which uses a modified VDRL antigen. Approximately 75 percent of patients with primary syphilis will have a positive VDRL (1), and all patients with secondary syphilis will have a positive serologic test for syphilis (STS). By definition latent syphilis will have a positive STS.

The FTA-ABS (fluorescent treponemal antibody absorption test) is the specific treponemal test for syphilis which has generally replaced the older *Treponema pallidum* immobilization (TPI) test and is the standard treponemal test in most state health laboratories. Results are ordinarily reported as reactive or nonreactive; reactivity is not quantitated. The FTA-ABS is more sensitive in all stages of syphilis than either the VDRL or the TPI. The VDRL is nonreactive in as many as one third of cases of late syphilis (2), and it is clearly necessary to perform the more sensitive FTA-ABS in any patient in whom there is clinical suspicion of late syphilis. Evidence for occasional false-positive FTA-ABS tests is slowly accumulating. This appears to occur most often in systemic lupus erythematosus (3). Pregnant women occasionally have false-positive FTA-ABS tests (4).

Blood specimens for diagnostic testing should first be subjected to a standard nontreponemal antigen STS. Nonreactive tests essentially exclude active syphilis except in the very early case. If the STS is reactive, a quantitative test should then be performed. A reactive serology verified by a second specimen in a patient in whom clinical and epidemiological evidence do not oppose the diagnosis means syphilis with a high degree of reliability. Biologic false-positive reactions do occur, however, and verification of a reactive nontreponemal antigen STS by the specific treponemal antigen test (FTA-ABS) is advisable. Specific treponemal antigen testing is imperative in individuals in whom clinical and epidemiologic evidence oppose the diagnosis of syphilis. A reactive FTA-ABS test when properly done indicates syphilis with as much reliability as serologic testing affords, though, as with any laboratory test, the result must be correlated with the clinical picture.

Epidemiologic Considerations

The physician's obligation is by no means completed when he diagnoses and treats his patient who has infectious syphilis. If control of syphilis is to be achieved, it is mandatory that the contacts, both source and possible spread, be examined. This may be taken care of entirely by the physician or assistance can be obtained from the local or state public health authorities who should be notified of the diagnosis in either case. If the patient's diagnosis is primary syphilis, all possible source contacts up to three months prior to the appearance of the lesion should be examined, and if secondary or early latent syphilis, for a six to twelve month period prior to diagnosis.

Whether to treat on a purely epidemiologic evidence or to follow the contact until a definite diagnosis is established or rejected is a problem which the private physician must handle on an individual basis. The promiscuous group or those difficult to follow are probably best treated on an epidemiologic basis once their initial examination has been completed and the serology drawn. If epidemiologic treatment is rejected, serologic testing should be continued for at least three months after the last sexual exposure.

While syphilis is transmitted primarily by heterosexual means, evidence is mounting that the homosexual male is considerably more promiscuous than the heterosexual male, and his role in the spread of venereal disease is rapidly increasing. The possibility of homosexual exposure must be considered in an increasing number of patients.

Treatment

Penicillin is the most effective antisyphilitic drug for the treatment of all stages of the disease. The results of treatment of early syphilis with penicillin are excellent by any standard. In a review of 636 patients, there was a cumulative retreatment rate of 4.4 percent, but in the majority retreatment was required because of reinfection rather than relapse or persistence of the original infection (5). The only serious problem is that of penicillin allergy which is reported variously as 0.8 percent to 5 percent (6, 7). To date, there has been no evidence of true resistance of *Treponema pallidum* to penicillin. When an infectious type of lesion appears after treatment, this is usually a manifestation of reinfection rather than relapse. Rigid differentiation between relapse and reinfection is often difficult or impossible.

In primary or secondary syphilis, or for prophylactic treatment of sexual contacts of syphilis, 2.4 million units of benzathine penicillin G (administered 1.2 million units in each buttock) is curative. Other acceptable schedules include aqueous procaine penicillin G, 600,000 units once daily for eight to ten days or procaine penicillin G with 2 percent aluminum monosterate in a dosage of 2.4 million units intramuscularly on the first day with an additional 1.2 million units on each of two subsequent injections three days apart. Recommended treatment for both early latent and late latent syphilis is 4.8 million units benzathine penicillin administered in two dosages of 2.4 million units seven days apart or aqueous procaine penicillin G, 600,000 units daily for ten days. In late syphilis including cardiovascular, neuro and visceral, benzathine penicillin G, 7.2 million units (2.4 million units weekly for three weeks) or aqueous procaine penicillin G, 600,000 units daily for fifteen days should be administered. Treatment of syphilis in pregnancy is the same depending on the stage; no additional medication is needed because of the pregnancy. Treatment of congenital syphilis is accomplished with a single injection of benzathine penicillin G in a dose of 50,000 units per kilogram of body weight.

Patients Sensitive to Penicillin

TETRACYCLINE: In infectious syphilis, tetracycline by mouth in a total dose of 30 grams administered over fifteen days is approximately as effective as penicillin (8). For latent syphilis, both early and late, the total dose should be 40 grams given 2 grams daily. Late syphilis requires at least 50 grams total dose. Because tetracycline may cause staining and other adverse effects on teeth and bones, it should not be used in pregnancy or in the treatment of patients less than six or seven years of age (9, 10).

DOXYCYCLINE: Doxycycline, one of the newer tetracyclines, has been evaluated in the treatment of early (infectious) syphilis and found effective when given orally 100 mgm twice daily for fifteen days. The chances of *missed medication* are probably much less on a twice daily schedule compared to a four times a day schedule (11).

ERYTHROMYCIN: Erythromycin estolate in a total dosage of 30 grams for infectious syphilis and both early and late latent syphilis is effective. For late syphilis (cardiovascular, central nervous system or visceral) a total dose of 40 grams administered 2 grams daily is required. Though it has no adverse effects on the fetus, erythromycin cannot be recommended for use in pregnancy because of reported failures to cure syphilis in utero (12, 13).

CEPHALORIDINE: Cephaloridine can be given with reasonable safety to the penicillin allergic patient and causes little pain upon injection. Clinical studies in early syphilis have shown that cephaloridine is effective in a dose of 0.5 grams daily for 10 days (14). Cephaloridine should be an excellent alternative to penicillin in penicillin allergic, pregnant patients with syphilis. Cephaloridine crosses the placenta to achieve levels in cord or fetal blood approximately 60 percent of those in the maternal circulation (15). Two cases of its successful use in pregnancy have been reported (16, 17). Moore has successfully employed cephaloridine using the schedule above in seven pregnant women who were allergic to penicillin (18).

Follow-up Study

The patient with primary or secondary syphilis should be followed clinically and with VDRL titers for one year at one, three, six and twelve-month intervals. The quantitative titer is the principal index for measuring therapeutic success. If the STS is still reactive at one year, the spinal fluid should be examined. In early latent and late latent syphilis post-treatment observation should include serologic follow-up at one, three, six and twelve-month intervals for the first year and then at six-month intervals for an additional year if the patient has not reverted to seronegativity. Thereafter a yearly STS for life is recommended once the VDRL has stabilized at a relatively low titer such as 1:4 or less. The spinal fluid need not be examined because it was necessarily normal to make the diagnosis of latent syphilis. The follow-up as outlined may be modified, especially if seronegativity is achieved.

Serologic response to treatment will vary according to the stage and duration of the disease. In general, a serologic cure will be achieved sooner in early syphilis than in latent or late syphilis. Almost all primary syphilis will be seronegative within six to nine months after treatment whereas about 95 percent of patients with secondary syphilis will be seronegative twelve months after treatment.

In late syphilis the serologic follow-up is the same as for latent syphilis. Titer of the reagin test will usually remain fixed or may diminish very slightly. It is extremely doubtful if any additional amount of antibiotics will further depress the serologic titer once an optimum dosage of antibiotic has been given. The FTA-ABS test can be expected to remain unaltered by therapy.

Therapy is considered a failure if any of the following supervenes: (a) infectious lesions do not heal or heal and reappear; (b) serologic titer does not diminish; (c) serologic titer falls and then rises *(serologic relapse)*. Distinction between failure and reinfection is often impossible. Retreatment may be performed with the same drug and dosage as the original treatment, keeping in mind the fact that a certain percentage of patients remain serofast regardless of treatment.

GONORRHEA

Introduction

Gonorrhea is the most prevalent of the venereal diseases and the most common bacterial infection of adults. The incidence of gonorrhea has risen steadily since 1958, and the number of cases reported annually has nearly doubled since 1965 (19). It is apparent that gonorrhea is undergoing rapid epidemiological as well as clinical changes. Asymptomatic gonorrhea in females is a phenomenon of the present outbreak; to a lesser extent asymptomatic gonorrhea also occurs in the male (20). One in ten women tested at some family planning clinics has asymptomatic gonorrhea (21). The reservoir of asymptomatic infections in females is a significant factor in the expanding pandemic occurring throughout the nation today and needs to be identified and treated. Serious clinical complications of gonorrhea especially in females are being encountered with increasing frequency. Questions regarding the possible effects of oral contraceptives upon gonorrheal infections have risen, however, for the most part they remain unresolved (22, 23).

Gonorrhea is no longer only a disease in the genitourinary tract of the male and female. The new sexual mores have led to gonococcal proctitis and gonococcal infection in the rectum. Gonococci have been isolated from the pharynx with increasing frequency and several cases of proven gonococcal pharyngitis have been reported (24, 25).

Bacteriology

The gonococcus is a delicate aerobic but facultative anaerobic organism, and culture isolation requires special media. Thayer-Martin medium is an antibiotic-containing medium selective for the pathogenic *Neisseria* (26). Recently this medium has been modified by the addition of more agar and dextrose and put up in screw-cap bottles containing 10 percent CO_2 to produce a transportable or mailable culture called Transgrow (27). The medium is commercially available. This enables all physicians to have good bacteriologic support available. When appropriate specimens are plated on Thayer-Martin medium or Transgrow and the resulting colonies have a colonial and microscopic morphology typical of *N. gonorrhea* and a positive oxidase reaction, the presumptive diagnosis of *N. gonorrhea* is virtually equivalent to a definitive diagnosis. Sugar fermentations should be performed for confirmation in cases of sexual assault, divorce or other medical-legal situations.

Clinical Disease

The risk of acquiring gonorrhea by contact with an infected female is estimated at 22 percent (28). In the male the usual incubation period is two to five days, however, this may be much longer (up to several weeks) or as short as twelve to twenty-four hours. Typically, patients have a sudden onset of frequent, painful urination accompanied by a discharge which is initially thin and watery but then rapidly becomes profuse and mucopurulent. Infection may progress to the posterior urethra, prostate, seminal vesicles or the epididymis.

In the female primary infection usually involves the cervix, ducts of Bartholin's glands, or periurethral ducts. Seventy-five to 90 percent of women with gonorrhea are asymptomatic. Only a small minority of women complain of vaginal discharge or have symptoms of urethritis. Profuse leukorrhea is rarely gonococcal in origin.

Gonococcal septicemia may result in several important clinical syndromes. Dissemination probably occurs more frequently in females because they are more often asymptomatic and untreated and therefore constitute the largest reservoir of gonococcal infection in the community. Male homosexuals with asymptomatic anorectal gonorrhea are analogous to the asymptomatic infectious females. A primary urogenital focus of infection may not be obvious since a significant number of patients with dissemination are asymptomatic (29). Careful bacteriologic studies will almost always yield a positive culture for *N. gonorrhea* from one or more sites.

Arthritis is the most frequently recognized manifestation of disseminated gonococcal infection. Gonococcal arthritis most commonly consists of a polyarticular arthritis or tenosynovitis involving knees, wrists, small joints of the hands, ankles and elbows. Less commonly monoarticular involvement occurs with significant effusion. Skin lesions are not uncommon and may be either hemorrhagic or vesiculopustular in type. The lesions are usually tender initially but then involute in three to five days even in the absence of treatment. The skin of the extremities, particularly the palms and soles and periarticular regions, are the sites of predilection. It is unusual to find gonococci in either a smear or a culture from one of these lesions.

Diagnosis

In the male the presence of gram negative intracellular diplococci in urethral pus together with typical clinical symptoms is virtually diagnostic. In cases of urethritis when the diagnosis is questionable or when there has been apparent treatment failure, culture on selective medium should be performed. Culture is also necessary to diagnose gonococcal proctitis or pharyngitis.

The diagnosis of gonorrhea in the female depends on cultural identification of the organism. Smears have no place in the diagnosis of gonorrhea in the female because of the very significant possibility of error in either direction. If only a single site is selected for culture, the cervix should be chosen since 85 to 90 percent of infected patients will harbor organisms at this site. Rectal cultures are positive in 30 to 50 percent of women with positive cervical cultures, and are positive by themselves in less than 10 percent. A negative culture does not rule out the diagnosis of gonorrhea because studies indicate that cultures from all four sites (cervix, rectum, urethra and vagina) will be negative in 6 to 8 percent of infected females at any one visit (30, 31). There is evidence which suggests that the diagnosis of gonorrhea may be facilitated in patients taking oral contraceptive agents because of more regular bacterial shedding (32). The specimen should be inoculated directly upon the medium because of the great susceptibility of the gonococcus to desiccation. If the inoculation has been made on Thayer-Martin medium, the inoculated plate should be promptly placed in a candle jar to retard drying and provide carbon dioxide. The use of the Transgrow medium makes this step unnecessary since the carbon dioxide is contained within the bottle.

Treatment

Gonococci which have greater resistance to penicillin than those seen prior to 1955 are emerging (33). Variations in the degree of resistance to penicillin are found in different geographic locales, and a treatment schedule reported as being of particular value in one area may not be the drug of choice elsewhere. Frequent local evaluation of treatment schedules is a necessity. In addition to resistance to penicillin, resistance is now developing to other antibiotics. Strains which have acquired penicillin resistance are more likely to have resistance to tetracycline (33). When penicillin resistance is present, tetracycline is unlikely to be of benefit. However, infections due to tetracycline-resistant gonococci are likely to respond to penicillin (34).

Despite the problem of resistance, penicillin remains the drug of choice in gonorrhea. Uncomplicated gonococcal urethritis in the male is adequately treated with 2.4 million units of aqueous procaine penicillin G in a single intramuscular injection. Females require higher doses to achieve the same satisfactory cure rate, and 4.8 million units of aqueous procaine penicillin G is recommended. The principle of therapy for gonorrhea is to obtain a high blood level of the antibiotic for a relatively short period, hence the use of the short acting penicillin. Benzathine penicillin or other long acting preparations, while ideal in syphilis, have no place in the treatment of gonorrhea. Patients failing to respond to this therapy should be retreated with twice the original amount over a two-day period. Male patients frequently complain of watery or mucoid discharge following therapy. This probably represents subsiding urethral inflammation and further therapy is generally not indicated unless it continues for more than five to seven days. Patients must be warned against self-examination and urethral stripping since this only prolongs the healing process.

Epididymitis or prostatitis ordinarily responds satisfactorily to 2.4 million units of aqueous procaine penicillin G daily for five to seven days. Acute gonococcal salpingitis requires high doses of procaine penicillin for seven to fourteen days.

Alternate Antibiotics

Patients who are allergic to penicillin may be treated with tetracycline. Most male patients will respond well to 3 or 4 grams given as an initial dose of 2 grams and the remainder in four hours. Women should receive 5 to 9 grams of tetracycline given as an initial dose of 2 grams followed by 0.5 gram four times daily.

Spectinomycin hydrochloride is a new parenteral antibiotic for treatment of gonorrhea. Several studies have now shown this to be extremely effective in doses of 2 or 4 grams in both men and women (35, 36).

Ampicillin is effective in 2.0 to 3.5 gram parenteral or oral single doses. When combined with oral probenicid, cure rates of 95 percent or better can be expected (37, 38, 39).

Cephaloridine in a 2.0 gram single dose results in somewhat higher failure rates than other alternate antibiotics (38, 40).

The significantly higher cost of both ampicillin and cephaloridine is not offset by a significantly higher therapeutic value, and it will be the unusual case of gonorrhea which warrants the additional cost of treatment with these agents.

Reexamination for determination of cure is generally not necessary in men since cessation of symptoms almost always indicates cure. However, in women reculture is essential for the proper management of gonorrhea. Follow-up cultures should be obtained one week following treatment and if possible again at two weeks. It has been suggested that gonococci in the rectum are more difficult to eradicate than gonococci at other sites (41, 42). However, we have not found this to be a problem (36).

As part of the complete therapy of the patient with gonorrhea it must not be forgotten that syphilis may have been contracted at the same time and from the source as the gonorrhea. Evidence has now been accumulated demonstrating that currently-recommended penicillin schedules for treatment of gonorrhea also cure incubating syphilis (34). Proper management of gonorrhea dictates that an initial serologic test be performed at the time the gonorrhea is diagnosed followed by monthly serologic tests for three months in all patients treated with alternate antibiotics.

REFERENCES

1. Wende, R. D., Mudd, R. L., Knox, J. M. and Holder, W. R.: The VDRL slide test in 322 cases of darkfield positive primary syphilis. *Southern Med J*, 64:633-634, 1971.
2. Harner, R. E., Smith, J. L. and Israel, C. W.: The FTA-ABS test in late syphilis. *JAMA*, 203:545-548, 1968.
3. Kraus, S. J., Haserick, J. R. and Lantz, M. A.: Fluorescent treponemal antibody absorption test reactions in lupus erythematosus: atypical beading pattern and probable false-positive reactions. *N Eng J Med*, 282:1287-1290, 1970.
4. Buchanan, D. S. and Haserick, J. R.: FTA-ABS test in pregnancy: probable false-positive reaction. *Arch Dermatol*, 102:322-325, 1970.
5. Jefferiss, F. J. G. and Wilcox, R. R.: Treatment of early syphilis with penicillin alone. *Br J Vener Dis*, 39:143-148, 1963.
6. Frank, P. F., Stollerman, G. H. and Miller, L. F.: Protection of a military population from rheumatic fever: routine administration of benzathine penicillin G to healthy individuals. *JAMA*, 193:775-783, 1965.
7. Minkin, W. and Lynch, P. J.: Incidence of immediate systemic penicillin reactions. *Milit Med*, 133:557-560, 1968.
8. Lucas, J. B. and Price, E. V.: Cooperative evaluation of treatment for early syphilis: preliminary report with special reference to spectinomycin sulfate (actinospectacin). *Br J Vener Dis*, 43:244-248, 1967.
9. Davis, J. S. and Kaufman, R. H.: Tetracycline toxicity: a clinico-pathologic study with special references to liver damage and its reference to pregnancy. *Am J Obstet Gynecol*, 95:523-529, 1966.
10. Kline, A. H., Blattner, R. J. and Lunin, M.: The transplacental effect of tetracycline on teeth. *JAMA*, 188:178-180, 1964.
11. Duncan, W. C., Knox, J. M. and Holder, W. R.: Treatment of early syphilis with doxycycline. *Br J Vener Dis*, In press.
12. South, M. A., Short, D. H. and Knox, J. M.: Failure of erythromycin estolate therapy in in utero syphilis. *JAMA*, 190:70-71, 1964.
13. Mamunes, P., Budell, J. W., Steward, R. E., Cave, V. G. and Anderson, J. A.: Early diagnosis of neonatal syphilis. *Am J Dis Child*, 120: 17-21, 1970.
14. Glicksman, J. M., Short, D. H. and Knox, J. M.: Parenteral cephaloridine treatment of patients with early syphilis. *Arch Intern Med*, 121:342-344, 1968.

15. Arthur, L. J. H. and Burland, W. L.: Transfer of cephaloridine from mother to fetus. *Arch Dis Child*, 44:82-83, 1969.
16. Flarer, F.: On the antitreponemic action of cephaloridine. *Postgrad Med J*, 43(suppl.):133-134, 1967.
17. Oller, L. Z.: Cephaloridine in gonorrhea and syphilis. *Br J Vener Dis*, 43:39-47, 1967.
18. Moore, M. B.: Personal Communication, 1970.
19. *Today's VD Control Problem—1971*. New York, American Social Health Association, 1971.
20. Pariser, H. and Marino, A. F.: Gonorrhea—frequently unrecognized reservoirs. *Southern Med J*, 63:198-201, 1970.
21. Allen, E. S.: Identification of the asymptomatic female carrier of *N. gonorrhoeae*. *Br J Vener Dis*, 46:334-335, 1970.
22. Juhlin, L. and Liden, S.: Influence of contraceptive gestogen pills on sexual behaviour and the spread of gonorrhea. *Br J Vener Dis*, 45: 321-324, 1969.
23. Cohen, L.: The "pill," promiscuity, and venereal disease. *Br J Vener Dis*, 46:108-110, 1970.
24. Fiumara, N. J., Wise, H. M. and Many, M.: Gonorrheal pharyngitis. *N Engl J Med*, 276:1248-1250, 1967.
25. Metzger, A. L.: Gonococcal arthritis complicating gonorrheal pharyngitis. *Ann Intern Med*, 73:267-269, 1970.
26. Thayer, J. D. and Martin, J. E.: Improved medium selective for cultivation of *Neisseria gonorrhoeae* and *Neisseria meningitidis*. *Public Health Rep*, 81:559-562, 1966.
27. Martin, J. E. and Lester, A.: Transgrow, a medium for transport and growth of *Neisseria gonorrhoeae* and *Neisseria meningitidis*. *HSMHA Health Reports*, 86:30-33, 1971.
28. Holmes, K. K., Johnson, D. W. and Trostle, H. J.: An estimate of the risk of men acquiring gonorrhea by sexual contact with infected females. *Am J Epidemiol*, 91:170-174, 1970.
29. Holmes, K. K., Counts, G. W. and Beaty, H. N.: Disseminated gonococcal infection. *Ann Intern Med*, 74:979-993, 1971.
30. Schmale, J. D., Martin, J. E. and Domescik, G.: Observations on the culture diagnosis of gonorrhea in women. *JAMA*, 210:312-314, 1969.
31. Caldwell, J. G., Price, E. V., Pazin, G. J. and Cornelius, C. E.: Sensitivity and reproducibility of Thayer-Martin culture medium in diagnosing gonorrhea in women. *Am J Obstet Gynecol*, 109:463-468, 1971.
32. Hewitt, A. B.: Oral contraception among special clinic patients with special reference to the diagnosis of gonorrhea. *Br J Vener Dis*, 46: 106-107, 1970.
33. Amies, C. R.: Sensitivity of *Neisseria gonorrhoeae* to penicillin and other antibiotics. *Br J Vener Dis*, 45:216-222, 1969.

34. Lucas, J. B.: Gonococcal resistance to antibiotics. *Southern Med Bull,* 59:22-28, 1971.
35. Cornelius, C. E. and Domescik, G.: Spectinomycin hydrochloride in the treatment of uncomplicated gonorrhea. *Br J Vener Dis,* 46:212-213, 1970.
36. Duncan, W. C., Holder, W. R., Roberts, D. P. and Knox, J. M.: Treatment of uncomplicated gonorrhea with spectinomycin hydrochloride: comparison with penicillin schedules. In preparation.
37. Kvale, P. A., Keys, T. F., Johnson, D. W. and Holmes, K. K.: Single oral dose ampicillin-probenicid treatment of gonorrhea in the male. *JAMA,* 215:1449-1453, 1971.
38. Keys, T. F., Halverson, C. W. and Clarke, E. J.: Single-dose treatment of gonorrhea with selected antibiotic agents. *JAMA,* 210:857-861, 1969.
39. Johnson, D. W., Kvale, P. A., Afable, V. L., Stewart, S. D., Halverson, C. W. and Holmes, K. K.: Single-dose antibiotic treatment of asymptomatic gonorrhea in hospitalized women. *N Engl J Med,* 283:1-6, 1970.
40. Lucas, J. B., Thayer, J. D., Utley, P. M., Billings, T. E. and Hackney, J. E.: Treatment of gonorrhea in males with cephaloridine. *JAMA,* 195:919-921, 1966.
41. Scott, J. and Stone, A. H.: Diagnosis of rectal gonorrhoea in both sexes using a selective culture medium. *Br J Vener Dis,* 42:103-106, 1966.
42. Schroeter, A. L. and Pazin, G. J.: Gonorrhea: diagnosis and treatment. *Ann Intern Med,* 72:553-559, 1970.

CHAPTER 3

THE ROLE OF IMMUNOGLOBULINS IN THE EARLY DIAGNOSIS OF CONGENITAL SYPHILIS

VERNAL G. CAVE

DUE APPARENTLY to the frequency and fury of treponemal showers or spirochaetemia, the earlier the stage of syphilitic infection in the pregnant female the greater is the possibility of congenital syphilis in the newborn. Ostensibly Langhans' layer of cells covering the chronic villi protects the fetus from treponemal infection during the first four months of pregnancy. After the 16th week of pregnancy with the progressive atrophying of Langhans' layer the fetus becomes vulnerable to infection. Recently, however, this traditional explanation of the reason why treponemal infection of the fetus does not occur early in pregnancy has been challenged, and the possibility of aspiration of infected amniotic fluid has been suggested. Whatever the mechanism, the fate of the infected fetus is influenced by several factors including the age of the fetus at the time of the infection and the number of infecting organisms. A great range of possibilities exists. These include the birth of an apparently normal infant whose infection may not become manifest until much later in life, premature delivery with manifest symptomatology or death of the fetus with maceration and spontaneous abortion.

The earlier the stage of the disease in the infected female, the greater is the possibility of infection of the fetus. Diagnosis of congenital syphilis at birth should not be difficult where there are manifest signs of congenital syphilis or where there is a significant titre elevation of a reactive cord serologic test in a neonate compared to the titration level of the mother utilizing conventional or nonspecific tests. The difficulty in diagnosis occurs when the only finding in the neonate is a reactive conventional serologic test which by maternal comparison is not significantly elevated in titre. The vast majority of these situations represents placental antibody transfer of maternal immunoglobulins, but which ones? The answer may be ascertained by serial testing using a conventional or nontreponemal serologic test such as the quantitative VDRL. The lowering and the eventual disappearance of these maternal antibodies will be reflected in progressively lower titration levels with reversal to nonreactivity in two to three months. Such a procedure runs a dual risk in infected neonates of further harm or of loss to follow-up. In many instances infants are treated without a definitive diagnosis and sometimes erroneously stigmatized.

In recent years it has been demonstrated that intrauterine infections will frequently result in abnormally elevated IgM levels. Much interest has been generated in the study of these immunoglobulins in cord or venous blood of neonates as a means of detecting prior intrauterine infection. In this connection a little background review may be useful.

TABLE 3-I

HUMAN IMMUNOGLOBULINS

Class	Sedimentation Constant	Approximate Mol. Weight	Serum Mg. Percent	Percent of Total Antibody Protein
IgG	7S	160,000	700 to 1500	At least 80
IgA serum (secretions)	7S, 11S, 18S	170,000	150 to 250	10
		600,000		
	11S	390,000		
IgM		900,000	60 to 170	5-10
IgD	7S	160,000	3	
IgE	8S	160,000	Very small	

The various proteins associated with antibody activity are referred to as immunoglobulins. Presently five main classes have been identified. They are IgG, or immunoglobulin G; IgA; IgM; IgD and IgE. Class IgG comprises at least 80 percent of the 7S immunoglobulins. The IgGs all have molecular weights approximating 160,000. Normal values are seven hundred to fifteen hundred milligrams percent.

Class IgA makes up about 10 percent of the immunoglobulins. Members of this class have varying molecular weights of from 170,000 to 600,000.

Class IgM immunoglobulins, of an approximate molecular weight of 900,000, account for 5 to 10 percent of the total antibody protein in serum.

Class IgD immunoglobulins which was discovered in the study of myeloma, comprise about 3 percent of immunoglobulins of normal sera and has a molecular weight in the neighborhood of 160,000.

Finally, class IgE isolated as a result of work on P-K antibody makes up a small but distinct class. It is present only in small amount and has a weight of about 160,000.

The high 900,000 molecular weight of IgM is of great importance in the study of intrauterine infections. The human placenta fairly readily permits the placental transfer of maternal globulins of Class IgG with its molecular weights in the neighborhood of 160,000 but will act as a barrier, not necessarily a purely mechanical barrier, but a barrier nonetheless to the transfer of maternal macroglobulins of Class IgM. However, the fetus is capable of elaborating macroglobulins of class IgM as an antigenic response to intrauterine infection. This response has been demonstrated in a number of intrauterine infections including rubella, cytomegalovirus inclusion disease, toxoplasmosis and syphilis. Elevated total IgM levels may be considered indicative of intrauterine infection of some kind. However, intrauterine infection, especially when not overwhelming, may not result in the presence of abnormally elevated total IgM levels at birth. It is, therefore, possible that the total IgM level of a neonate infected in utero with rubella may be 20 milligrams percent or less, which is in the normal range. Consequently, it is not surprising that interest has been generated in identifying specific IgM antibodies to specific diseases within the total IgM complex. Indeed work has been done in this area in syphilis as well as other diseases including the ones referred to above.

In 1966 Deacon, Lucas and Price described the Fluorescent Treponemal Antibody Absorption test (FTA-ABS). Deacon and his associates used a stable, water soluble extract of Reiter treponeme (sorbent) to absorb from test serum common antibodies which *Treponema pallidum* shares with such nonpathogenic treponemes as *Treponema microdentium* and the Reiter treponeme. The antigen used in the FTA-ABS test is a lyophilized virulent *Treponema pallidum* of the Nichols strain produced in the same manner as for the *Treponema pallidum* immobilization test described by Nelson and Mayer in 1949. A suspension of these organisms is allowed to air dry in a thin smear on a glass slide and is affixed with acetone. Following this a 1:5 dilution of test serum is added to the smear. If the patient's specimen contains human antitreponemal antibody, globulin will adhere to the treponeme, producing an antigen-antibody complex. It is now necessary to demonstrate that this reaction has taken place. The first antigen-antibody complex now acts as an antigen. The treponeme coated with human globulin is the new antigen. A conjugate consisting of anti-IgG antibody linked with fluorescein is now added to the slide. A second antigen-antibody complex is produced which on examination under an ultraviolet microscope will show fluorescence. This FTA-ABS test, has to this point, essentially stood the test of time.

In 1968 Scotti and Logan, in a preliminary study, announced an experimental indirect fluorescent antibody test for demonstrating IgM immunoglobulins specific for *T. pallidum*. Scotti and Logan modified the FTA-ABS test as just described by Deacon and his associates. Scotti and Logan's one modification of this test was to substitute antihuman IgM conjugated with fluorescein for the fluorescein tagged antihuman or anti-IgG antibody. Scotti and Logan found their test to be reactive in all three cases of proved syphilis and to be nonreactive in ten cases of clinically negative infants with reactive VDRL and FTA-ABS tests. In addition, six clearly nonsyphilitic infants were nonreactive in all tests. They cautioned, however, that the sensitivity of the test could not be determined from their study. In 1969, Alford, Polt, Cassady and others working at the Alabama Medical Center reported a comparative study using the gamma-M-FTA-ABS, routine FTA-ABS, the gamma-G-FTA-ABS, the VDRL and total serum gamma-M levels in eight infants with different clinical forms of syphilis. They concluded that the gamma-M-FTA-ABS test was superior to any other test known to that time for the early diagnosis of congenital syphilis. So satisfied were they with the results of the gamma-M-FTA-ABS test that it has been incorporated as a standard serologic procedure in their hospital's diagnostic laboratory. However, in that same report they cautioned that with the use of an extract of Reiter treponeme small amounts of specific antibody may be removed. They suggested the use of Evans blue for dilution, but here again caution that, although this procedure may increase sensitivity in the specimen, specificity may be decreased.

In 1968 Mamunes, Cave and others began a cooperative study by the New York City Department of Health and the Department of Pediatrics of the New Jersey College of Medicine and Dentistry. They attempted to identify the presence of antitreponemal IgM antibodies using a different modification of the standard FTA-ABS test than was used by Scotti and Logan. In this study, phosphate-buffered saline was used as the diluent in place of sorbent because of the unlikelihood of fetal exposure to the nonpathogenic treponemes and because it was known that sorbent reduces the sensitivity of the test. Commercial fluorescein tagged antihuman IgM antibody was substituted for the fluorescein tagged antihuman globulin and used in a dilution sufficient to eliminate nonspecific staining of control nonreactive sera and yet give a 4+ reaction in known reactive sera.

The results suggested that the gamma-M-FTA test as performed in that study may be sensitive enough to detect all infants born with congenital syphilis whether symptomatic or asymptomatic.

Levels of IgM of 20 milligrams percent or less in neonates at birth are considered normal. In this study cord levels of IgM in the cases of active disease ranged from 7 to 276 milligrams percent. We concluded that total IgM determinations under these circumstances are not reliably elevated in cases of congenital syphilis.

To date, the largest series of cases aimed at identifying specific IgM in the diagnosis of neonatal congenital syphilis was reported by Scotti, Logan and Caldwell in 1969 on 149 specimens. Their studies, however, did not reveal any cases in which their experimental tests were reactive at birth in infants who were asymptomatic at birth and could not be diagnosed as congenital syphilis using conventional criteria. They concluded that the IgM-FTA-ABS test, "Although useful as it is presently performed, should be considered an experimental procedure until its sensitivity can be established."

Continued studies utilizing the IgM-FTA with any particular modification have been inhibited in recent times by inability to obtain a suitable antihuman IgM fluorescein conjugate. However, recently the Public Health Service by cooperation and encouragement has been able to identify three commercial sources from which antihuman IgM conjugate may be obtained both for the purpose of diagnostic and necessary experimental studies. These companies are as follows:

1. Wellcome Reagents,
   Division Burroughs Wellcome Co.
   3030 Cornwallace Road
   Research Triangle Park, North Carolina 27709
2. Canalco, Inc.
   5635 Fisher Lane
   Rockville, Maryland 20852
3. Kallestad Laboratory, Inc.
   4005 Vernon Avenue
   Minneapolis, Minnesota 55416

This information, however, does not constitute endorsement by the P.H.S. or myself.

Now that reliable antihuman IgM conjugate is available, all laboratories presently equipped to do the Fluorescent Treponemal Antibody Absorption Test can perform IgM-FTA tests by simple modification and although this test must still be considered experimental, it is indeed possible to develop over the next few years a body of evidence which will be able to define more

TABLE 3-II

REACTIVITY OF VDRL, FTA-ABS AND TPI TESTS DURING
VARIOUS STAGES OF SYPHILIS*

Category	Number Tested	Percent Reactive		
		FTA-ABS Test	TPI Test	VDRL Test
Primary	191	85	56	78
Secondary syphilis	270	99	94	97
Late syphilis	117	95	92	77
Latent syphilis	954	95	94	74
Presumably normal	384	1	0	0

* Data adopted from tables presented by Deacon and others.

precisely the role of a standard IgM-FTA test in the early diagnosis of congenital syphilis. This can be done by the careful examination of infants with reactive IgM-FTA Tests at birth who are followed closely for a sufficient period of time. Table II will show what may be anticipated with the FTA-ABS test. One notes here that the FTA-ABS test becomes positive earlier in syphilis than any other serologic test for syphilis and remains reactive for longer periods of time. One also notes that the FTA-ABS test is reactive in primary syphilis in 85 percent of cases as opposed to a much lower percentage for the TPI and the VDRL and in late syphilis is 95 percent reactive whereas the TPI and the VDRL are only 77 percent reactive. The FTA-ABS test may persist reactive for many years even after adequate therapy. One can postulate that if a reactive FTA-ABS test in the neonate is due to passive transfer of antibodies that six, nine, twelve and twenty-four months later no passively transferred antibodies will be demonstrable by this test. Likewise, if the patient has a persistently positive FTA-ABS test, the specificity of the IgM-FTA test done at birth may be verified.

IN CONCLUSION

As of this date the IgM-FTA test must be considered as still experimental. However, the following points may be made:

1. Total IgM level (20 milligrams or less being normal), although helpful in the diagnosis of intrauterine infection, is not reliably elevated in all cases of intrauterine infection and certainly is not indicative of a specific intrauterine infection.

2. The various modifications of the IgM-FTA test indicate that there is a strong possibility of defining an additional reliable tool in the diagnosis of congenital syphilis at birth.

3. The tendency of the FTA-ABS test to persist reactive for long periods of time and sometimes for life despite adequate therapy provides an excellent opportunity for retrospective evaluation of any prospective study.

4. The identification by the Public Health Service of three sources for obtaining antihuman IgM conjugate provides an excellent opportunity for widespread performance of this test in neonates with reactive conventional serologic tests. The opportunity now exists for the accumulation of a body of evidence within the next several years to devise a reliable standard technique using fluorescent procedures for the identification of specific IgM immunoglobulins in the early diagnosis of congenital syphilis in neonates at birth.

CHAPTER 4

EVALUATION OF TREATMENT FOR EARLY SYPHILIS

ARNOLD L. SCHROETER

MORE THAN A QUARTER of a century has now passed since penicillin was first used for the treatment of syphilis by Mahoney and others (1). Penicillin and other antibiotics have replaced arsenical and heavy metal therapy. Subsequently, the general use of antibiotics precipitated a rapid drop in the incidence of infectious syphilis in the early 1950's. However, the number of reported cases of infectious syphilis escalated from 6,251 in 1957 to 23,750 cases in 1965. With the continuous rise in the incidence of syphilis in 1965, reassessment of treatment schedules recommended by the U.S. Public Health Service (USPHS) for early syphilis was deemed essential. Although no antibiotic resistance of *Treponema pallidum* had been noted or reported, during the 1950's the accelerated resistance of the gonococcus to penicillin was well documented. Furthermore, the recommended treatment schedules in the United States had been employed without reevaluation since the determination of their efficacy in the late 1940's and early 1950's.

In the 1950's alternate antibiotics, other than penicillin, were evaluated and found to be efficacious in the treatment of syphilis. Tetracycline and erythromycin, because of their usefulness, were established as excellent alternates for penicillin in the treatment of syphilis. Consequently, the USPHS, until 1965, recommended a ten-day treatment with oral doses of tetracycline or erythromycin in a total dosage of 30 and 20 gm, respectively. The initial evaluation of erythromycin was made with erythromycin estolate (2). Based on these evaluations, 20 gm of erythromycin given over ten days was recommended for the treatment of early syphilis. Because of reports of cholestatic hepatitis after the use of erythromycin estolate, other analogues, including the base form of erythromycin, were being used for such treatment.

In July 1965 the Venereal Disease Branch of the Center for Disease Control initiated an evaluation to establish the current comparative efficacy of schedules now recommended by the USPHS for the treatment of patients having early stages of syphilis. Physicians in nine metropolitan areas (Los Angeles, Washington, D.C., Miami, Detroit, New York, Philadelphia, El Paso, Houston and Norfolk) agreed to participate in the evaluation. In addition to antibiotic efficacy, we will report the comparative serologic treatment response to the following tests: Venereal Disease Research Laboratory (VDRL), fluorescent treponemal antibody absorption (FTA-ABS), and the *T. pallidum* immobilization (TPI) tests.

MATERIALS AND METHODS
Selection of Cases and Examination of Patients

Selection of patients was limited to those with dark-field, positive lesions of primary or secondary syphilis with either initial infection or reinfection.

The initial examination of the patients, in addition to the dark-field, included a complete physical examination and a serologic test for syphilis. Whole blood specimens taken at examinations both before and after treatment were submitted to the Center for Disease Control, Venereal Disease Research Laboratory, Atlanta, for the VDRL, FTA-ABS, and TPI tests. Follow-up after treatment included physical examination and serologic tests scheduled monthly for the first year and quarterly for the second year. Only one spinal fluid examination was requested in cases of treatment failure or at the end of the two year observation period.

Criteria for Cure

The criteria for cure depended on the disappearance of clinical manifestations and on prompt and permanent decreased titer of the VDRL quantitative test. Relapse was determined clinically by the reappearance of lesions and by a significant and sustained increase in VDRL test titer. In addition, failure of serologic titer to respond significantly during the first year after treatment was defined as treatment failure. Reinfection, although difficult at times to differentiate from relapse, was epidemiologically identified whenever possible.

Treatment Schedules

Six schedules of treatment were employed in the evaluation as follows: (a) benzathine penicillin G—single injection 2.4 million units; (b) procaine penicillin G in oil—total 4.8 million units (2.4 million units at first session and 1.2 million units at each of two subsequent sessions at three-day intervals); (c) aqueous procaine penicillin G—600,000 units daily for total of 4.8 million units; (d) tetracycline (orally)—total 30 gm (3 gm/day for ten days); and (e) erythromycin (orally)—total 20 gm (2 gm/day for ten days). Later a 30-gm schedule of erythromycin was used. All drugs were secured by the venereal disease program and distributed to cooperating clinics so that identical preparations could be evaluated by the participants. At the end of the first year of study it was evident that the base form of erythromycin, when administered in a dosage of 20 gm, was inadequate therapy for early syphilis. At the time the inadequacy of the erythromycin schedule was determined, a preliminary report was made (3). Limited data then indicated that the majority of treatment failures occurred in patients who were receiving less than 300 mg/kg of body weight. The 20-gm schedule, therefore, was discontinued, and a 30-gm schedule was substituted. The cooperating clinics were instructed to re-treat all patients whose course was not completely satisfactory subsequent to use of the 20-gm erythromycin schedule.

RESULTS

Each of the 584 patients admitted to the study was placed on one of the six treatment schedules. Attempts were made to follow the condition of all patients according to the planned schedule for twenty-four months; however, the final follow-up was completed in only 146 cases. To make adjustments for the pro-

TABLE 4-I

EARLY SYPHILIS: CUMULATIVE RE-TREATMENT RATE*

Observation After Treatment (Mo.)	Benzathine Penicillin G, 2,400,000 U (100 Pt.)		Procaine Penicillin G in Oil, 4,800,000 U (101 Pt.)		Aqueous Procaine Penicillin G, 4,800,000 U (61 Pt.)		Tetracycline, 30 gm (107 Pt.)		Erythromycin 30 gm (144 Pt.)		Erythromycin 20 gm (71 Pt.)	
	No. of Pt. Observed	Cum Percent Re-Treated	No. of Pt. Observed	Cum Percent Re-Treated	No. of Pt. Observed	Cum Percent Re-Treated	No. of Pt. Observed	Cum Percent Re-Treated	No. of Pt. Observed	Cum Percent Re-Treated	No. of Pt. Observed	Cum Percent Observed Total
3	90	0.0	85	3.3	58	0.0	99	1.0	126	2.4	61	3.3
6	75	3.4	71	3.3	52	3.8	87	5.3	102	4.1	51	18.3
9	62	3.4	61	3.3	46	3.8	75	7.8	85	8.3	45	24.4
12	55	5.1	54	3.3	41	3.8	67	9.2	68	10.9	38	26.8
15	55	5.1	53	3.3	37	3.8	62	10.8	63	14.1	37	26.8
18	45	7.3	43	7.9	34	3.8	52	12.7	38	14.1	33	29.9
21	34	7.3	34	10.9	26	3.8	48	12.7	30	14.1	26	29.9
24	25	11.4	28	10.9	15	10.7	40	12.7	14	21.3	23	29.9

* Includes both reinfection and treatment failures.

gressive loss of patients from observation, the statistical method described by Iskrant and others for evaluating antisyphilitic therapy was used in this study (4).

The cumulative re-treatment rate, including both treatment failure and reinfection, is shown in Table 4-I. The re-treatment rate of the first twelfth-month observation is weighted less by re-infections than is the rate at the twenty-fourth month. At the twelfth month follow-up, re-treatment rates for the penicillin schedules ranged from 3.3 percent after 4.8 million units of procaine penicillin G in oil to 5.1 percent after 2.4 million units of benzathine penicillin G, or an average of 4.0 percent. Re-treatment rates for the tetracycline schedule at twelve months were significantly higher (9.2 percent) than average penicillin re-treatment rates ($P = 0.05$). Excluding erythromycin at the twenty-fourth month of observation, the re-treatment rates ranged from 10.7 percent for aqueous procaine penicillin G to 12.7 percent for tetracycline. At twenty-four months of follow-up the failure rate (12.7 percent) for the tetracycline schedule was not significantly different from the penicillin schedules.

At the twelfth month of follow-up, the re-treatment rates for the 30-gm and 20-gm erythromycin schedules were 10.9 and 26.8 percent, respectively. The 20-gm erythromycin schedule continued to have a high failure rate (29.9 percent) through the twenty-fourth month. The large increase in the rate of the 30-gm treatment schedule at the twenty-fourth month is due to the small number of cases observed and a single reinfection at this period.

A more detailed analysis of the two erythromycin schedules may be made from Table 4-II, which differentiates therapy relapse from reinfection. If reinfection is distinguished from relapse, the 30-gm erythromycin schedule at the twelfth month of observation demonstrated significantly better efficacy than did the 20-gm schedule.

A complete analysis of the data is precluded by the relatively small number of cases; however, the analysis of efficacy of treatment by body weight dosages and sex of patients may be helpful in confirming the efficacy of the larger dose schedule of erythromycin. In Figure IV-1, which shows the cumulative re-treatment

TABLE 4-II

COMPARATIVE EFFECTIVENESS OF ERYTHROMYCIN (BASE) IN TREATMENT OF EARLY SYPHILIS
(NO HISTORY OF SYPHILIS OR PREVIOUS TREATMENT)

Observation After Treatment (Mo.)	Erythromycin (Base Form)							
	20-gm Schedule				30-gm Schedule			
	No. of Patients Observed	Cumulative Percent Re-Treated			No. of Patients Observed	Cumulative Percent Re-Treated		
		Total	Relapse	Rein-fection		Total	Relapse	Rein-fection
Primary Syphilis								
3	35	5.7	5.7	0.0	72	4.2	1.4	2.7
6	27	19.7	13.0	6.7	56	5.7	1.4	4.2
9	21	19.7	13.0	6.7	47	7.6	1.4	6.1
12	19	24.7	13.0	11.7	39	9.9	3.7	6.1
15	17	24.7	13.0	11.7	37	9.9	3.7	6.1
18	13	24.7	13.0	11.7	21	9.9	3.7	6.1
21	*	..	..	..	17	9.9	3.7	6.1
24	*	..	..	..	*	..	..	..
Secondary Syphilis								
3	26	0.0	0.0	0.0	41	0.0	0.0	0.0
6	24	16.4	12.4	4.0	33	2.6	0.0	2.6
9	24	29.0	25.0	4.0	30	12.3	3.2	8.0
12	20	29.0	25.0	4.0	22	16.5	3.2	12.2
15	20	29.0	25.0	4.0	19	16.5	3.2	12.2
18	20	34.1	25.0	9.1	11	16.5	3.2	12.2
21	17	34.1	25.0	9.1	*	..	..	..
24	14	34.1	25.0	9.1	*	..	..	..
Total								
3	61	3.3	3.3	0.0	113	2.7	0.9	1.8
6	51	18.3	12.8	5.5	89	4.6	0.9	3.7
9	45	24.4	18.9	5.5	77	9.4	2.1	7.3
12	39	26.8	18.9	7.9	61	12.3	3.5	8.8
15	37	26.8	18.9	7.9	56	12.3	3.5	8.8
18	33	29.9	18.9	11.0	32	12.3	3.5	8.8
21	26	29.9	18.9	11.0	25	12.3	3.5	8.8
24	23	29.9	18.9	11.0	10	22.0	3.5	18.5

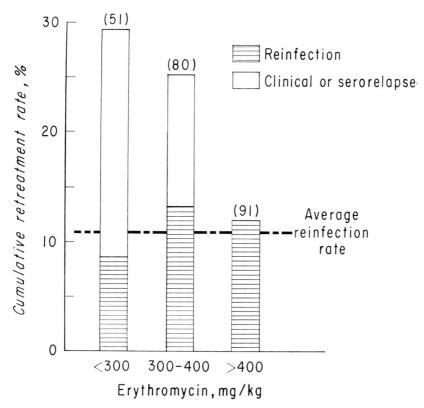

Figure IV-1. Cumulative rate for erythromycin base re-treatment after 15 month of observation by milligram per kilogram of body weight.

rate after fifteen months of observation by milligram per kilogram of body weight, the reinfection rate remained fairly constant (varying from 8.6 to 12.2 percent), but the therapy relapse rate dropped from 21 percent in patients treated with less than 300 mg/kg of body weight to 0 percent in patients receiving more than 400 mg/kg.

When sex as well as body weight is considered, as in Figure IV-2, both factors apparently influence results. Because of the small number of cases, males have been divided into two groups —those receiving more and those receiving less than 350 mg/kg of body weight. These two groups are compared with the total number of females treated. Approximately two thirds of the fe-

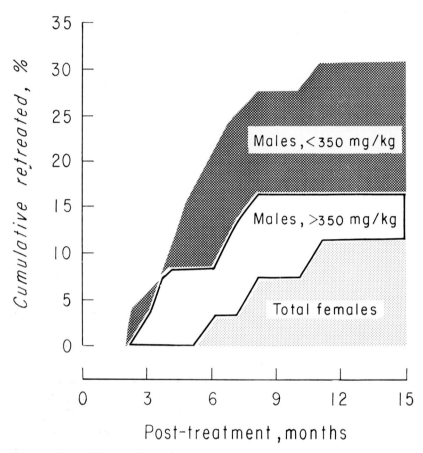

Figure IV-2. Efficacy of erythromycin base for the treatment of syphilis for males and females based on milligrams per kilogram of body weight.

males received more than 300 mg/kg. In addition, the condition of two thirds of the females was diagnosed as secondary syphilis. In contrast, 58 percent of the males had primary syphilis and were treated with less than 350 mg/kg. In the male group treated with more than 350 mg/kg, 74 percent had primary syphilis. This distribution should favor greater efficacy of therapy in the males; however, the reverse was true.

Table 4-III suggests that erythromycin is less effective treatment for males than for females. If this difference was strictly a matter of taking oral medication as prescribed, the difference in sex would be observed for all oral therapy. Although the re-treatment rates for penicillin and tetracycline are equivalent for males and females, this is not true for erythromycin. The re-treatment rate for males is twice that for females. A possible explanation for this difference may be that severe gastrointestinal disturbances were much more frequent with erythromycin (6 percent) than with tetracycline (1 percent). Males treated with 30 gm of erythromycin not only reported more reactions but also necessitated the termination of treatment more frequently than males treated with tetracycline. In fact, 10.5 percent of patients taking erythromycin terminated treatment because of reaction in comparison with 1 percent of patients taking tetracycline. Furthermore, among the 24 males who required re-treatment, at least four later admitted that they failed to complete treatment with erythromycin or they prolonged treatment beyond the prescribed ten days.

In Figure IV-3 the proportion of re-treatment rates that were attributed to relapse or to reinfection is shown for each schedule for the twelfth, eighteenth and twenty-fourth months of observation. When patients with previous infections were added, the re-treatment rate for benzathine penicillin G and tetracycline showed the greatest increase because these two schedules were most frequently used as re-treatment schedules. Except for the 20-gm dosage of erythromycin, treatment failure rates for all therapy schedules were less than 4 percent, and reinfection contributed to the major portion of the re-treatment rates.

TABLE 4-III

COMPARISON OF MALE AND FEMALE RE-TREATMENT RATES
FOR EARLY SYPHILIS

| | | *Males* | | | *Females* | |
| | *Total* | *Re-treated* | | *Total* | *Re-treated* | |
Drug	*No.*	*No.*	*Percent*	*No.*	*No.*	*Percent*
Penicillin (i.m.)	188*	10	5.3	46	2	4.3
Tetracycline (orally)	39	5	12.8	26	2	7.7
Erythromycin (orally) ...	159	24	15.1	36	3	8.3

* Crude rates unadjusted for patients lost from observation.

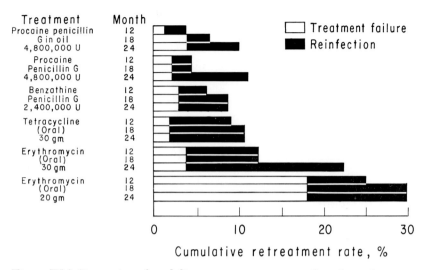

Figure IV-3. Proportion of syphilis re-treatment rates attributed to relapse or to reinfection shown for each schedule. The graph is limited to previously untreated patients.

Excluding the unsuccessful 20 gm erythromycin schedule, the differences between re-treatment rates of the successful individual schedules at twelve months were not significant.

Serologic Tests Results

The analysis of serologic test results is limited to patients receiving penicillin, tetracycline and 30 gm of erythromycin (Table 4-IV) by stage of syphilis. No significant difference could be found among reinfection rates as reported by stage of syphilis. No treatment failures occurred in primary syphilis with nonreactive VDRL tests. In primary and secondary syphilis with reactive VDRL tests at the twenty-fourth month of observation, the treatment failure rates were 2.7 percent and 4.4 percent, respectively. In primary syphilis, with reactive VDRL tests, 17 percent of the cases were still reactive at the twelfth month and 2.8 percent at more than two years. In secondary syphilis the reactivity rate was 49 percent at twelve months and 11.6 percent at more than two years.

In addition to stage of syphilis, the height of the VDRL quantitative titer seemed to influence the speed at which sero-

TABLE 4-IV

RESULTS OF TREATMENT BY STAGE OF EARLY SYPHILIS: TOTAL OF FIVE RECOMMENDED SCHEDULES (INITIAL INFECTIONS ONLY)

Seronegative primary syphilis

Observation After Treatment (Mo.)	No. of Patients Observed	Cumulative Percent Re-treated			Not Re-treated, Percent	
		Total	Relapse	Reinfection	Seroreactive	Serononreactive
	60					
3	56	0.0	0.0	0.0	8.9	91.1
6	49	1.9	0.0	1.9	4.1	94.0
9	40	1.9	0.0	1.9	0.0	98.1
12	31	4.6	0.0	4.6	0.0	95.4
15	31	4.6	0.0	4.6	0.0	95.4
18	25	8.6	0.0	8.6	0.0	91.4
21	22	8.6	0.0	8.6	0.0	91.4
24	11	8.6	0.0	8.6	0.0	91.4
> 24	8	8.6	0.0	8.6	0.0	91.4

Seropositive primary syphilis

Observation After Treatment (Mo.)	No. of Patients Observed	Cumulative Percent Re-treated			Not Re-treated, Percent	
		Total	Relapse	Reinfection	Seroreactive	Serononreactive
	213					
3	185	3.2	0.5	2.6	75.7	21.1
6	156	5.6	1.1	4.4	42.4	52.0
9	135	6.3	1.1	5.1	25.8	67.9
12	120	7.9	2.7	5.1	16.6	75.6
15	114	7.9	2.7	5.1	15.8	76.4
18	82	7.9	2.7	5.1	8.5	83.7
21	66	7.9	2.7	5.1	9.1	83.1
24	47	10.0	2.7	7.2	4.3	85.8
> 24	36	10.0	2.7	7.2	2.8	87.2

Secondary syphilis

Observation After Treatment (Mo.)	No. of Patients Observed	Cumulative Percent Re-treated			Not Re-treated, Percent	
		Total	Relapse	Reinfection	Seroreactive	Serononreactive
	176					
3	159	0.6	0.6	0.0	98.8	0.6
6	128	3.4	2.1	1.3	81.1	15.6
9	110	7.7	3.0	4.8	63.4	29.0
12	95	8.7	3.0	5.8	49.4	42.0
15	87	8.7	3.0	5.8	38.9	52.6
18	72	11.5	4.4	7.2	38.8	49.9
21	54	13.3	4.4	9.0	29.6	57.3
24	38	15.9	4.4	11.6	23.7	60.5
> 24	30	15.9	4.4	11.6	23.6	60.6

Total primary and secondary syphilis

Observation After Treatment (Mo.)	No. of Patients Observed	Cumulative Percent Re-treated			Not Re-treated, Percent	
		Total	Relapse	Reinfection	Seroreactive	Serononreactive
	449					
3	400	1.7	0.5	1.3	75.5	22.8
6	333	4.2	1.4	3.0	51.7	44.2
9	285	6.3	1.7	4.7	36.8	57.1
12	247	7.8	2.5	5.4	27.1	65.2
15	233	7.8	2.5	5.4	22.3	70.0
18	180	9.5	3.1	6.5	19.5	71.2
21	142	10.2	3.1	7.2	15.5	74.5
24	96	12.3	3.1	9.3	11.5	76.4
> 24	73	12.3	3.1	9.3	11.0	76.9

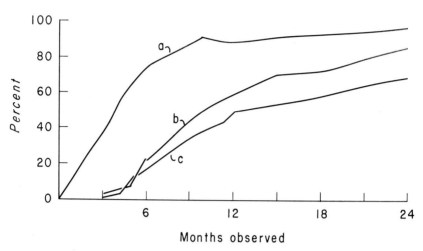

Figure IV-4. Comparison after treatment of serologic reactivity of syphilitic patients with titers of less than 1:8 (a), of 1:16 to 1:32 (b) and of 1:64 (c).

negativity was achieved. In Figure IV-4 values for seronegativity obtained at each observation after therapy for patients with titers of 1:8 or less, 1:16 to 1:32 and 1:64 or more are compared. In these three groups the percentages of patients with secondary syphilis were 7, 62 and 72 percent, respectively. In the low titer group 74 percent of the patients were nonreactive by the sixth month after treatment. In patients with titers of 1:16 to 1:32 only 50 percent had reverted by the tenth month of observation, and approximately twenty months elapsed before 75 percent had obtained seronegativity. It required more than a year for the majority of patients with titers of 1:64 or more to become nonreactive and more than 30 percent of this group still maintained a low titer after two years of observation.

Eighty patients, adequately treated and observed for two years, had FTA-ABS, TPI and VDRL tests on pretreatment specimen and on specimens obtained at six, twelve and twenty-four months of observation (Fig. IV-5). The VDRL slide test became nonreactive most rapidly with weak reactions predominating from the sixth month on. Weak reactions were reported in two thirds of the patients still showing reactivity at the twenty-fourth month of observation. The TPI test, which had the lowest pretreatment reactivity rate, showed definite response to treatment. The FTA-ABS test, which had the highest reactivity rate before treatment (96 percent), showed no particular response during the first year of observation. At the twenty-fourth month 78 percent of the patients were still reactive and another 16 percent had borderline reaction; that is, 94 percent still showed some reactivity.

A group of 208 patients was tested by the FTA-ABS and VDRL tests before treatment and at the sixth and twelfth months of observation. At twelve months' observation 23 patients (11 percent) had a nonreactive FTA test. All 23 patients had primary syphilis; 12 of these 23 had a nonreactive VDRL test before treatment. Only one patient who had a VDRL titer of more than 1:8 had a nonreactive FTA-ABS test after treatment.

The response of the FTA-ABS test after adequate treatment is shown in Figure IV-6 by stage of syphilis. In patients with primary syphilis and a nonreactive VDRL test, the reactivity rate of the FTA-ABS test dropped in twelve months from 78 percent prior to treatment to 28 percent or to 33 percent if borderline results were included. In patients with a reactive VDRL test and primary syphilis the reactivity rate dropped from 97 percent to

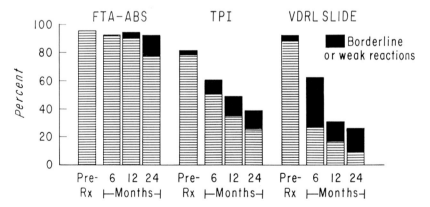

Figure IV-5. Comparison of results of serologic reactivity of 80 patients observed for 2 years with the FTA-ABS, TPI and VDRL tests.

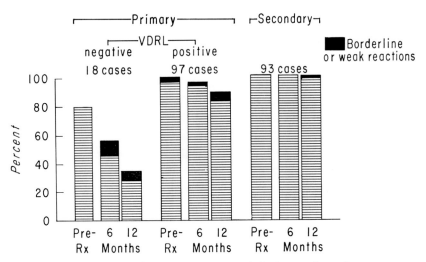

Figure IV-6. Response of 208 patients to FTA-ABS test after adequate treatment. Observed for 12 months.

83 percent or from 99 percent to 89 percent if borderline results are included. Although borderline results are not reported by the laboratory as reactive, in observations after treatment they do complete the picture.

Reaction to Treatment

Reactions to treatment ranged from 1.6 percent of patients treated with benzathine penicillin G to 14 percent of patients treated with 30 gm of erythromycin. Twelve patients (12/335, or 3.6 percent) reported reactions to penicillin. Among patients treated with the various penicillin schedules, those treated with aqueous procaine penicillin G had the highest rate of reactions (8.6 percent), but the only anaphylactic reaction followed the administration of crystalline penicillin G in 2 percent aluminum monostearate in oil (PAM). Urticaria, angioneurotic edema and pruritus were the principal reactions to penicillin. Moderate to severe gastrointestinal disturbances occurred in 2.3 percent of the patients treated with tetracycline and in 11.3 percent of patients treated with erythromycin.

COMMENT

Penicillin remains the drug of choice for the treatment of patients with early syphilis. In this study no detectable change could be demonstrated in the therapeutic efficacy of penicillin G for the treatment of early syphilis as compared with earlier studies in the late 1950's (5-9). When the results of this study are compared to those of Smith and others no significant differences were detected despite minor changes in amount and frequency of penicillin administered (9). The cumulative re-treatment rate for all penicillin schedules for primary syphilis in our study was 7.5 percent as compared to 4.0 percent in Smith and associates' evaluation of 2.5 million units of benzathine penicillin G. In secondary syphilis our cumulative re-treatment rate was 11.9 percent and in Smith and associates' evaluation 5.5 percent for 2.5 million units of benzathine penicillin G. Furthermore, when the results of this study are compared with the study of Capinski and others in 1968 (10), the serologic responses for primary and secondary syphilis are comparable. In the study of Capinski and others nonreactive VDRL status had developed in 42 percent of patients treated for secondary syphilis by the time of the two-year follow-up; in comparison, 60 percent of the patients with secondary syphilis similarly followed in this study became nonreactive. These treatment results confirm the unpublished work of Clark (11) who did not demonstrate significant change in the amount of penicillin needed to cure rabbits infected with fresh human strains of *T. pallidum*.

Four types of erythromycin are currently used for therapy: erythromycin base, erythromycin estolate, erythromycin stearate and erythromycin ethyl succinate. Of the four, erythromycin estolate is uniquely absorbed. Chemically, the estolate form is the lauryl sulfate propionyl ester of erythromycin. Erythromycin estolate, in comparison with the base form, has greater stability and gastrointestinal absorption. Consequently, the estolate form produces the highest blood level of all the erythromycin analogues; that is, taken orally, 250 mg of the estolate compound results in an earlier rise to the same blood concentration with the same duration as that with 1,000 mg of erythromycin base (12). In addition, gastrointestinal complications are rare after the intake of erythromycin estolate, since it has less influence on intestinal bacterial flora than do the other forms of erythromycin.

The initial studies evaluating the efficacy of erythromycin in the treatment of syphilis were performed using erythromycin estolate. These studies showed that 15 or 20 gm of erythromycin estolate was adequate for treatment of early syphilis (2). On the basis of these studies, the USPHS recommended that for early syphilis 20 gm of erythromycin be given over ten days. However, due to the possible complications of cholestatic hepatitis associated with the taking of erythromycin estolate (13), the recommendations at that time did not specify the form of erythromycin to be used. Since erythromycin base produced a lower blood level, the efficacy was predictably less than the estolate for the treatment of early syphilis if equivalent dosages were compared. This study showed this conclusively. A 25 percent re-treatment rate was obtained with the 20-gm schedule of erythromycin in comparison with a rate of 9.9 percent obtained with the 30-gm schedule after a twelve-month follow-up. Based on these results, a minimal dosage of 30 gm of erythromycin is recommended for the treatment of early syphilis.

The reason for the excessively high failure rate of 20 gm of the erythromycin base form may be related not only to the absorption pattern but also to the influence of body weight dosage. As expected, more severe gastrointestinal disturbances were caused by treatment with erythromycin base than with tetracycline. For this reason, many of the male patients discontinued their therapy, whereas the female patients, despite possible gastrointestinal upset, continued to take their medication. The fortitude of the females to continue to take their medication may have produced a lower treatment failure rate of 8.3 percent compared to the rate of 15.1 percent in the males. Despite the gastrointestinal side effects, the base form of erythromycin administered in a dosage of 30 gm (minimum, 400 mg/kg of body weight) over ten days was proved to be an acceptable alternative for penicillin in the treatment of early syphilis.

South and others (14) and Mamunes and others (15) reported

a treatment failure in a case of syphilis and pregnancy. In the case reported by South and others (14) a pregnant patient was treated with 15 gm of erythromycin estolate; an infant was born with signs of congenital syphilis and died during the third day of life. The most likely reason for erythromycin treatment failure in this case could have been due to inadequate placental transfer of erythromycin. The concentration of erythromycin as reported in the fetal serum is only $\frac{1}{6}$ to $\frac{1}{16}$ that in the maternal serum (16-18). Therefore, a low dose of erythromycin may effect inadequate low concentrations in the fetal tissue. On the other hand, the expected failure rate of erythromycin for the treatment of syphilis is 12.3 percent, which includes cases of therapy failure as well as reinfection. Therefore, these two cases may fall within the expected number of treatment failures or reinfections and do not prove inadequacy of erythromycin to cure syphilis in pregnancy. Retrospective analysis of previous syphilis therapy studies documents five cases of syphilitic pregnancies in which treatment utilizing recommended erythromycin dosages was adequate with no evidence of congenital syphilis in the infant (2).

The only alternative to treating a pregnant patient who has penicillin allergy would be to utilize tetracycline. Tetracycline, in the dosage required to treat syphilis, however, most certainly would cause mottling and staining of fetal dentition and possibly abnormal formation of bone (19). Furthermore, the cord blood concentrations of tetracycline are approximately $\frac{1}{2}$ to $\frac{1}{16}$ that of maternal blood (20, 21), which is only slightly better placental antibiotic transfer than with erythromycin. In light of the fact that erythromycin given in adequate dosages is adequate treatment for early syphilis, it would appear that this drug would be a more acceptable alternative treatment for syphilis in pregnancy. Notwithstanding the necessity for maximal dosages of erythromycin to ensure adequate concentration in fetal tissue, additional studies are needed to establish efficacy of erythromycin for the prevention of congenital syphilis.

On the whole, the tetracycline group comprises essentially the five analogues that are closely related. They all give comparable therapeutic results. This is particularly true with their antisyphilitic effect. The first antibiotic of the tetracycline group to be used for the treatment of syphilis was chlortetracycline, which was found to be effective by O'Leary and others (22). Since then other analogues of the tetracycline group have been evaluated and found to be equally effective. The dosage is the same for all five compounds, namely a total of 30 gm equally distributed over a period of ten days (23). The results of this study confirm those in earlier reports suggesting that there has been no change in efficacy of tetracycline for the treatment of syphilis.

In all cases in this study patients were given standard serologic tests for syphilis so that adequate serologic response to treatment could be documented and serologic test response to treatment could be studied. The earlier adequate treatment is applied in the course of syphilitic infection, the sooner seronegativity may be obtained. In the five successful treatment schedules used, serum became reactive after treatment in only 9 percent of patients with primary syphilis and nonreactive VDRL tests, but after six months all returned to seronegativity. In the VDRL tests, serologically reactive primary syphilis became reactive in 87.2 percent of the patients who had nonreactive VDRL test results at the end of twenty-four months of observation as compared to 60.5 percent who had secondary syphilis.

The response of the serologic test is dependent not only on the stages of the disease but also on the height of the titer before treatment. The lower the VDRL test titer, the more quickly and the more frequently seronegativity may be obtained (Fig. IV-4). Patients with a titer of less than 1:8 return to seronegativity more rapidly than those with a higher titer, and at the twenty-four-month observation a greater percentage were seronegative as compared to those with titers of 1:16 to 1:32.

The FTA test was found to be the most sensitive test in all stages of syphilis. This was especially true in those patients who had dark-field positive primary syphilis but had nonreactive VDRL tests. In primary syphilis with reactive VDRL tests the FTA-ABS test responded with a decrease in reactivity from 97 to 83 percent. However, by the time secondary syphilis developed the FTA-ABS test did not show response to treatment within a twelve-month period. When all patients treated for early syphilis were grouped together and compared, the FTA test was the least responsive to treatment as compared with the TPI or the VDRL test. Thus the high sensitivity of the FTA-ABS test makes it an excellent diagnostic tool, but confirms the principle that the VDRL slide test should be used after treatment to document adequacy of therapy.

CONCLUSIONS

Since penicillin G was first instituted as therapy for the treatment of early syphilis there has been no detectable change in its efficacy. The results of use of tetracycline (30 gm given over a ten-day period) compared favorably with those of other recommended penicillin schedules. The base form of erythromycin, when administered in a dosage of no less than 30 gm (minimum of 400 mg/kg of body weight) over a period of ten days, is an acceptable alternative for penicillin in the treatment of early syphilis. Although the most sensitive serologic test for syphilis, the FTA-ABS test showed a definite decrease of reactivity after treatment of primary syphilis. The FTA-ABS test having the highest reactivity rate before treatment in all stages of syphilis responded more slowly to therapy than either the VDRL or the TPI test.

REFERENCES

1. Mahoney, J. F., Arnold, R. C. and Harris, A: Penicillin treatment of early syphilis: a preliminary report. *Vener Dis Inform*, 24:355-357, 1943.
2. Brown, W. J., Simpson, W. G., Moore, M. B., *et al.*: Oral propionyl erythromycin in treating early syphilis. *Public Health Rep*, 78:911-917, 1963.
3. Lucas, J. B. and Price, E. V.: Co-operative evaluation of treatment for early syphilis: preliminary report with special reference to spectinomycin sulfate (actinospectacin). *Br J Vener Dis*, 43:244-248, 1967.
4. Iskrant, A. P., Bowman, R. W. and Donohue, J. F.: Technique in evaluation of rapid antisyphilitic therapy. *Public Health Rep*, 63:965-983, 1948.
5. Idsøe, O., Guthe, T., Christiansen, S., *et al.*: A decade of reorientation in the treatment of venereal syphilis. *Bull WHO*, 10:507-561, 1954.
6. Smith, C. A. and Price, E. V.: American experience with penicillin alone in the treatment of syphilis. In Hellerström, S., Wekström, K. and Hellerström, A. M. (eds.): *Proceedings of the 11th International Congress of Dermatology*. Lund, Hikan Ohlssons Boktryckeri, 1960, vol. III, p. 896-903.
7. Smith, C. A., O'Brien, J. F., Simpson, W. G., *et al.*: Treatment of early

infectious syphilis with n,n'dibenzylethylenediamine dipenicillin G. *Am J Syph*, 38:136-142, 1954.

8. Shafer, J. K. and Smith, C. A.: Treatment of early infectious syphilis with n,n'-dibenzylethylenediamine dipenicillin G: a second report. *Bull WHO*, 10:619-626, 1954.

9. Smith, C. A., Kamp, M., Olansky, S., *et al.*: Benzathine penicillin G in the treatment of syphilis. *Bull WHO*, 15:1087-1096, 1956.

10. Capinski, T. Z., Lebioda, J., Kolasa, B., *et al.*: Antibiotics in the treatment of early syphilis. *Curr Probl Dermatol*, 2:39-51, 1968.

11. Clark, J. W.: Personal communication.

12. Griffith, R. S. and Black, H. R.: A comparison of blood levels after oral administration of erythromycin and erythromycin estolate. *Antibiot Chemother* (Basel), 12:398-403, 1962.

13. Braun, P.: Hepatotoxicity of erythromycin. *J Infect Dis*, 119:300-306, 1969.

14. South, M. A., Short, D. H. and Knox, J. M.: Failure of erythromycin esolate therapy in in utero syphilis. *JAMA*, 190:70-71, 1964.

15. Mamunes, P., Cave, V. G., Budell, J. W., *et al.*: Early diagnosis of neonatal syphilis: evaluation of a gamma M-fluorescent treponemal antibody test. *Am J Dis Child*, 120:17-21, 1970.

16. Heilman, F. R., Herrell, W. E., Wellman, W. E., *et al.*: Some laboratory and clinical observations on a new antibiotic, erythromycin (Ilotycin). *Proc Staff Meet Mayo Clin*, 27:285-304, 1952.

17. Keating, W. J. and Chesley, R. F.: Erythromycin and carbomycin: evaluation in treatment of puerperal infections. *Bull Margaret Hague Matern Hosp*, 7:46-48, 1954.

18. Henderson, F. G., Powell, C. E., Rose, C. L., *et al.*: Pharmacodynamics of Ilotycin (erythromycin, Lilly) (abstract). *J Pharmacol Exp Ther*, 106:395, 1952.

19. Demers, P., Fraser, D., Goldbloom, R. B., *et al.*: Effects of tetracyclines on skeletal growth and dentition: a report by the nutrition committee of the Canadian Paediatric Society. *Can Med Assoc J*, 99:849-854, 1968.

20. Maynard, A. L., Andriola, J. C. and Prigot, A.: Tetracycline hydrochloride studies on absorption, diffusion, excretion, and clinical trial. In Welch, H. and Martí-Ibáñez, F. (eds.): *Antibiotics Annual 1953-1954*. New York, Medical Encyclopedia, Inc., 1953, p. 102-107.

21. Milberg, M. B., Kamhi, B. and Banowitch, M. M.: Pharmacology and therapeutic efficacy of tetracycline. *Antibiot Chemother*, 4:1086-1099, 1954.

22. O'Leary, P. A., Kierland, R. R. and Herrell, W. E.: The oral administration of Aureomycin (duomycin) and its effect on Treponema pallidum in man. *Proc Staff Meet Mayo Clin*, 23:574-578, 1948.

23. Montgomery, C. H. and Knox, J. M.: Antibiotics other than penicillin in the treatment of syphilis. *N Engl J Med*, 261:277-280, 1959.

CHAPTER 5

THE EFFECTS OF GONORRHEA THERAPY ON INCUBATING SYPHILIS

James B. Lucas

SINCE 1961 THE Venereal Disease Branch of the United States Public Health Service has conducted an extensive series of studies relating to the therapy of incubating syphilis.

In the years prior to 1965 two cooperative clinical evaluations were carried out basically to determine the minimal dosages of antibiotics necessary to abort incubating syphilis. These studies were important since it had become apparent in the early 1960's that the control of infectious syphilis would require extensive epidemiologic treatment of those persons exposed to early lesion syphilis (1, 2, 3). It was hoped that these initial studies would demonstrate the complete efficacy of either relatively small doses of penicillin or an alternate antibiotic in aborting incubating syphilis, and permit a recommendation for epidemiologic treatment apart from that recommended in early syphilis.

The first of these studies was presented in 1963 by Moore, Price, Knox and Elgin (4) while a subsequent extension of this initial study remained unpublished. In both these studies patients were included who were clinically and serologically negative, but who had been exposed to infectious syphilis within a preceding 90 day period. Four drug schedules were included in the initial study, three of which consisted of single doses of penicillin. The schedules were benzathine penicillin G (Bicillin) in doses of 600,000 and 2.4 million units; aqueous procaine penicillin G (APPG), 600,000 units and 500 mgs of tetracycline giv-

71

en on two consecutive days, totaling 1 gram. A fifth group was given placebo treatment and served as the control. All patients were followed for at least three months with biweekly physical examinations and monthly serologic tests.

It was found that 9.2 percent of the control patients developed syphilis. The 600,000 unit dose of benzathine penicillin was 84 percent protective and the same dose of APPG only 46 percent protective. No patient receiving 2.4 million units of benzathine penicillin developed syphilis. The tetracycline schedule had no effect in preventing the disease. Both the APPG and tetracycline schedules appeared to slightly prolong the incubation period with 66 percent and 36 percent respectively of the failures not becoming apparent until the third month. This contrasts with the control group where 94 percent of infections were noted within the first 60 days. This study established that 2.4 million units of benzathine penicillin would abort all cases of incubating syphilis, an expected finding since this dosage had been recommended for the treatment of primary or secondary syphilis since 1955.

Since it was still hoped that some lower dosage might be recommended for epidemiological treatment, the study was continued. A benzathine penicillin G schedule of 1.2 million units was added as were 1 and 2 gram injections of chloramphenicol. A procaine penicillin G in oil with aluminum monostearate (PAM) schedule of 1.2 million units was also included. This PAM schedule was then the recommended standard and widely used treatment for gonorrhea. A composite of the results obtained in these two studies is presented in Table 5-I. The 1.2 million unit doses of benzathine penicillin and the PAM schedule were both quite effective, but still some 5 percent less effective than 2.4 million units of benzathine penicillin. The chloramphenicol schedules were only about 50 percent effective and the tetracycline group faired only slightly better than the controls, 10.9 percent of whom developed syphilis. From these studies it was concluded that not less than 2.4 million units of benzathine penicillin G could be completely relied upon in epidemiologic treatment. Since the PAM gonorrhea treatment schedule did not prevent all cases of syphilis, a four-month period of serologic

TABLE 5-I

EFFECTS OF VARIOUS ANTIBIOTIC SCHEDULES IN ABORTING
INCUBATING SYPHILIS
(Persons Exposed Within Preceding 90 Days)

Type and Amount of Treatment	Total Cases Treated	Observed	Developed Syphilis Number	Cum. Percent	Relative Efficacy (Percent)
Benzathine—2.4 MU	222	209	0	0.0	100.0
PAM*—1.2 MU	242	225	1	0.5	95.0
Benzathine—1.2 MU	212	194	1	0.7	94.0
Benzathine—0.6 MU	153	140	2	1.5	86.0
APPG—0.6 MU	150	134	5	4.2	61.0
Chloromycetin—1 Gm	101	96	4	5.1	53.0
Chloromycetin—2 Gms	37	35	2	6.0	45.0
Tetracycline—1 Gm	142	127	11	9.6	12.0
PLACEBO	393	375	38	10.9	0.0
Total	1,652	1,535	64	4.6	

* PAM—Procaine penicillin in oil with 2 percent aluminum monostearate.

follow-up continued to be recommended for gonorrhea patients (5). This recommendation was continued after the widespread adoption of APPG in gonorrhea therapy (6).

Beginning in 1963-64 the number of strains of *Neisseria gonorrhoeae* being received at the Venereal Disease Research Laboratory for penicillin sensitivity testing began showing rather marked increases in *in vitro* resistance. For the first time isolates were encountered which required one or more units of penicillin for inhibition. Realizing that the emergence of these resistant strains would probably require modification of the current therapy for gonorrhea a series of investigations was undertaken by the late Dr. James D. Thayer and his associates at the Venereal Disease Research Laboratory. Working in the Atlanta Federal Penitentiary with volunteers, men were infected with gonococcal isolates having known degrees of penicillin resistance and then treated with various types and doses of penicillin. It was found that when men were infected with isolates requiring 0.2 to 0.3 unit of penicillin for *in vitro* inhibition, consistent *in vivo* cure required large doses of short-acting penicillins. Preparations like benzathine penicillin G or PAM had little effect and produced low cure rates in these patients (7).

In addition to these studies a survey of routine, unselected, gonococcal isolates was carried out for the first time in 1965. This survey revealed that nearly one half of the isolates showed some degree of resistance to penicillin and that about 5 percent were actually resistant to 0.5 unit of penicillin or more (8).

Based on the human inoculation studies, as well as the survey results, the Public Health Service, in 1965, began to recommend 2.4 million units of APPG for males with gonorrhea and double this amount in females (6). When a patient had also been exposed to syphilis an additional injection of 2.4 million units of benzathine penicillin was also recommended since the effects of 2.4 million units of APPG on incubating syphilis were unknown.

While the earlier study by Moore and others (4) utilizing 600,000 units of APPG suggested that larger amounts might prove somewhat more effective certain earlier studies in the literature suggested that large doses of APPG might be very effective.

As early as 1945, Magnuson and Eagle had studied the time-dose relationships in experimental rabbit syphilis (9). In one experiment they demonstrated that 400 units of crystalline penicillin given every three hours for five doses would abort rabbit syphilis for up to forty-eight hours after an inoculation of 2,000 organisms. Longer incubation resulted in an increasing failure rate. It was shown that where penicillin failed to prevent the appearance of the primary lesion it regularly caused a significant prolongation of the incubation period. In other experimental studies it was shown that early syphilis in animals could be cured with aqueous penicillin administered for twelve, eighteen, twenty-four and forty-eight hours, respectively (10, 11). R. C. Arnold is cited in Moore's book *Penicillin in Syphilis* (12) as having demonstrated cures in fully established lesion animal syphilis in as short a time as twelve hours using enormous doses equal to 28 million units for a 70 Kg man.

In 1952 Arnold, Cutler, Wright and Levitan (13) reported retreatment rates of 0, 12.7 and 33.2 respectively for cases of seronegative primary, seropositive primary and secondary syphilis using a single injection of 300,000 units of PAM. In that same year Hollander (14) in a series of elegant animal experiments was able, using sodium penicillin G in subcurative doses, to prolong the incubation period of experimental syphilis in direct relationship to the dose size up to a limit of thirty to forty days. He did not observe wholly symptomless infections when the incubation period was prolonged. That is, the animals were either cured or developed clinically recognizable lesions. The good results in seronegative primary syphilis with 300,000 units of PAM were confirmed in 1955 by Cutler, Olansky and Price (15). These results were interpreted to mean that the then standard gonorrhea treatment of 600,000 units of PAM was adequate to abort any incubating syphilis that might be coexistent.

The switch in 1965 from the much longer acting PAM to the short acting APPG in gonorrhea therapy again raised the question of the effects on incubating syphilis. The duration of blood levels resulting from the 2.4 and 4.8 million unit doses of APPG were unknown, although they were assumed to be substantially longer than the twenty-four hour span seen with more conventional doses.

Prior to testing the effects of the newly recommended gonorrhea schedules in patients exposed to syphilis, a preliminary study in rabbits was undertaken. Care was taken to simulate insofar as possible the most likely sequence of events in coexposure to both gonorrhea and syphilis.

Materials and Methods

Twenty-eight young male rabbits were inoculated intradermally with 10^2 to 10^3 Nichols' strain virulent *T. pallidum* at six separate skin sites. All animals were bled prior to inoculation and the serum stored for serologic testing.

Sixteen animals were treated with aqueous procaine penicillin G on a weight basis corresponding to a dose of 4.8 million units for a 70 Kg human. Treatment was given on the sixth day following infection, an interval corresponding to a period in which 85 percent of men acquiring gonorrhea would have become symptomatic. To determine the minimal penicillin exposure time required for cure the treated animals were divided into four equal groups, three of which were given injections of 200,000 units of penicillinase at six, nine and twelve hours respectively following penicillin treatment to destroy any circulating penicillin. Serum was collected thirty minutes after the penicillinase injection and assayed for residual penicillin. The remaining group received no treatment other than penicillin.

Twelve animals served as various controls. These consisted of three groups of four animals. One group received no treatment of any kind. One group received daily injections of 200,000 units of penicillinase for ten days. The final group received a daily injection of 0.2 ml of a penicillin-penicillinase admixture for ten days. This mixture was prepared by reacting *in vitro* 3 million units of APPG with 800,000 units of penicillinase at 36°C for four hours. Assay of this mixture revealed only .034 unit/ml of inhibitory substance.

All animals were observed daily for chancre development. Suspicious areas were repeatedly examined by dark-field microscopy. All animals were bled at six and ten weeks post-inoculation. The VDRL slide agglutination test was performed on both pre- and post-inoculation sera. One animal died on the ninth day, three days following penicillin therapy.

After a four-month observation period lymph node transfers were carried out using an equal number of seronegative young male rabbits. The recipient animals were examined physically and serologically as previously described.

Results

Of the 15 surviving penicillin treated animals none developed chancres. Thirteen of the 15 remained serologically negative. One animal was found to have a false positive reaction which declined from a pre-inoculation titer of 1:1 to weakly reactive at ten weeks. The other animal had a nonreactive prebleeding but was weakly reactive at six and ten weeks. This reactivity may have been in response to the antigenic stimulus of the inoculum, but the *spontaneous* development of weakly reactive serologies in rabbits is not unusual. Serum assays failed to detect residual penicillin in those groups which received penicillinase.

In the group of 12 control rabbits all but one developed dark-field positive chancres. This single animal, who was in the daily penicillinase group, also failed to develop a reactive serology and evidently was not infected by the means employed. A single animal which developed dark-field positive lesions remained sero-nonreactive at ten weeks. All other 10 control rabbits developed reactive serologies, the average titer being 1:4 at six weeks and 1:8 at ten weeks.

The incubation period for the control animals developing dark-field positive lesions ranged from twenty to twenty-seven days with a mean of twenty-three days. There was no significant difference in the incubation time for the three control groups and none was expected since penicillinase has no known anti-treponemal activity. The mean incubation period corresponded closely to that observed in human cases. These data are summarized in Table 5-II.

The results of lymph node transfers confirmed the original observations. All recipient rabbits of penicillin-treated donors remained clinically and serologically negative, confirming that biologic cure had taken place. Recipients of tissue from untreated control rabbits all developed clinical and/or serologic evidence of syphilis, as expected.

This preliminary study established that in the animal model single large doses of APPG, comparable to a weight basis to that used in treating human gonorrhea were able to completely abort incubating syphilis when allowed to act for as short a time as six hours.

Based upon these highly suggestive animal experiments a third cooperative clinical study was developed. The logistics of this study were similar to the previous studies discussed with the ex-

TABLE 5-II

THE EFFECT OF APPG ON INCUBATING SYPHILIS IN RABBITS

	Penicillin Treated	Controls
Number*	15	12
Dark-field positive	0	11
Serology reactive	2†	10

* Number completing observation period.
† One false reactor and one weakly reactive.

ception that only patients who had been named as contacts to infectious syphilis within the preceding thirty days were included. This change was made to eliminate the follow-up of large numbers of patients whose last exposure was already well beyond the average incubation period and who had little likelihood of being infected. Venereal disease clinics in eight cities, Atlanta, Baltimore, Chicago, Dallas, Louisville, Milwaukee, Newark and New York, participated in the study which was begun in 1967 and not finally completed or analyzed until early 1971.

Methods

All patients were volunteers who had been named as sexual contacts to known cases of infectious syphilis and who had been exposed within the preceding thirty days. Only patients without clinical or serologic evidence of syphilis were included and they were randomly assigned to one of five major groups. One group received 2.4 million units of benzathine penicillin and served as a positive control. A dose of 2.4 million units of APPG was given to males as a single injection and 4.8 million units in a divided dose was given to females. A fourth group received one and a half grams of tetracycline orally in a single dose with another one and a half grams given six hours later, a total dose of 3 grams. The placebo group received an injection of sterile saline. One participating clinic used 2.4 million units of PAM in males and 3.0 million units of PAM in females. These two schedules corresponded to the routine therapy for gonorrhea then employed in that facility.

Quantitative VDRL slide tests were obtained at least monthly and biweekly physical examinations were carried out for a minimum of three months following therapy. Dark-field examinations were performed on suspicious lesions when noted. Patients developing syphilis were immediately treated with 2.4 million units of benzathine penicillin G.

Upon completion data cards were forwarded to the Venereal Disease Branch for tabulation and statistical analysis. Analysis of therapy results were performed in the manner of Iskrant and others (16, 17).

Results and Discussion

A composite of the results are found in Table 5-III. A total of 400 patients entered the study and 373 completed at least three months of follow-up. None of the patients treated with penicillin developed syphilis, while 30.3 percent in the placebo group developed the disease. The results with the 2.4 and 4.8 million unit doses of APPG are highly significant, when compared with the placebo group ($P < .001$). While the total number of patients receiving either of the two PAM schedules separately is too small for analysis the outcome for the combined PAM group is significantly better than the placebo group ($P < .05$). The difference observed between the 1.5 and 3.0 gms tetracycline schedules is not significant; nor are the outcomes between the placebo group and the 1.5 gms tetracycline or combined 1.5 and 3.0 gms tetracycline groups significantly different. However, the results with the 3.0 gms tetracycline schedule is significantly better than the placebo ($P < .05$). The group receiving 2.4 million units of APPG faired significantly better than either the 1.5 or 3.0 gms tetracycline schedules (P values $< .01$ and $< .05$ respectively).

TABLE 5-III

RELATIVE EFFICACY OF VARIOUS SCHEDULES OF
THERAPY IN ABORTING INCUBATING SYPHILIS
(Persons Exposed within Preceding 30 Days)

Treatment	Total Cases Treated	Observed[†]	Developed Syphilis Number	Percent	Relative Efficacy (Percent)
Benzathine—2.4 MU	84	79	0	0.0	100.0
APPG*—4.8 MU	72	66	0	0.0	100.0
APPG—2.4 MU	55	51	0	0.0	100.0
PAM‡—2.4 MU	13	10	0	0.0	100.0
PAM—3.0 MU	11	9	0	0.0	100.0
Tetracycline—3.0 Gms	76	73	9	13.3	56.0
Tetracycline—1.5 Gms	28	28	6	22.1	27.0
PLACEBO	61	57	16	30.3	0.0
Total	400	373	31	9.0	

* Aqueous procaine penicillin G.
† Minimum 90 days of follow-up.
‡ Procaine penicillin G in oil with 2 percent aluminum monostearate.

TABLE 5-IV

INITIAL DIAGNOSTIC CATEGORIES OF PLACEBO
AND THERAPY FAILURE PATIENTS

Therapy	Primary	Secondary	Early Latent	Total
Placebo	16	12	9	37
Benzathine Pen. 1.2 MU	1	0	0	1
PAM 1.2 MU	0	0	1	1
Chloromycetin 1 Gm	3	0	1	4
Chloromycetin 2 Gms	2	0	0	2
Tetracycline 1.5 Gms	1	0	5	6
Tetracycline 3 Gms	6	0	3	9
Total	29	12	19	60

It is difficult to assess from our data whether or not subcurative therapy prolonged the incubation period or masked the development of symptoms since only 23 patients have been therapeutic failures in the combined data for the last two cooperative studies. Other investigators have encountered the same problem (18, 19). It is worth noting, however, that about one third of the placebo group was diagnosed as secondary cases when first detected (Table 5-IV), but that this diagnosis was never made in the group receiving subcurative therapy. Similarly, only 9 of the 37 (24 percent) placebo cases had proceeded to latency before detection while 10 of 23 (44 percent) of the therapy failures were initially diagnosed as latent. This suggests that subcurative therapy may well mask or modify the natural course of syphilis.

Prolonged follow-up might be required to absolutely ascertain the efficacy of therapy in incubating syphilis. Previous studies (18, 19) have utilized an eighteen-month follow-up period. Today, however, long periods of post therapy follow-up have become impractical, despite the additional validity gained by longer observation. With longer follow-up periods reinfection becomes more of a problem than long term relapse.

Summary and Conclusions

The foregoing data present the efforts of the Public Health Service during the last decade to directly measure the effects of gonorrhea treatment schedules on incubating syphilis. Indirectly, an approach to this problem may be made by retrospective analysis of venereal disease clinic records, i.e. examining the records of early syphilis patients for previous gonorrhea therapy within the critical period or conversely by searching gonorrhea records to ascertain the subsequent development of syphilis. Obviously, since dual infections are a function of the incidence of both diseases within a given population and since reported gonorrhea cases far out number syphilis an analysis of this type requires a great number of accurate records and a relatively stable clinic clientele. Recently a survey of this type was reported from England by Woodcock (21) who felt that no proven conclusions could be arrived at using this approach. His findings did indicate that preceding penicillin therapy for gonorrhea did not influence the stage of early syphilis subsequently diagnosed and that penicillin given for gonorrhea is more likely to cure incubating syphilis than to mask it.

On the basis of the data presented, it is felt that the following conclusions and recommendations can be made:

1. Exposure to early infectious syphilis carries a substantial risk of infection which fully justifies the universal adoption of epidemiological treatment.

2. The gonorrhea schedules of 2.4 and 4.8 million units of APPG, as recommended for males and females, is completely adequate to abort incubating syphilis. Neither a serologic follow-up for syphilis nor additional treatment for gonorrhea patients who are sexual contacts to infectious syphilis is indicated.

3. Broad spectrum antibiotics in single session or short courses frequently used for the treatment of gonorrhea are inadequate to abort incubating syphilis in a high percentage of cases. Patients so treated should be followed with three monthly serologic tests.

4. Penicillin sensitive gonorrhea patients who are treated with broad spectrum antibiotics and who are also contacts to infectious syphilis should receive a full ten-day, 30-gram course of erythromycin or tetracycline to insure the abortion of incubating syphilis until further study indicates that less therapy is sufficient to accomplish this goal.

REFERENCES

1. Allison, J. R., Jr.: Epidemiological treatment of syphilis. *J SC Med Assoc*, 6:239-241, 1965.
2. Dougherty, W. J.: Epidemiological treatment of syphilis contacts. *J Med Soc NJ*, 59:564-566, 1962.

3. Editorial: Epidemiological treatment of syphilis. *JAMA*, 188:820, 1964.
4. Moore, B. M., Jr., Price, E. V., Knox, J. M. and Elgin, L. W.: Epidemiologic treatment of contacts to infectious syphilis. *Public Health Rep*, 78:966-970, 1963.
5. U.S. Public Health Service: Notes on Modern Management of VD. PHS Publication No. 859, U.S. Government Printing Office, Washington, D.C., p. 16-17, 1964.
6. Ibid. Gonorrhea, interim recommended treatment schedules. July 1965.
7. Thayer, J. D., Schroeter, A., Martin, J. E., Jr., Peacock, W. L., Jr. and Samuels, S. B.: Relationship of Penicillin-Resistant Gonococci to Failure in the Penicillin Therapy of Gonorrhea. Abstracts of the Fourth Interscience Conference on Antimicrobial Agents and Chemotherapy, 1964, p . 2-3.
8. Martin, J. E., Jr., Lester, A., Price, E. V. and Schmale, J. D.: Comparative study of gonococcal susceptibility to penicillin in the United States, *J Infect Dis*, 122:459-461, 1970.
9. Magnuson, H. J. and Eagle, H.: The retardation and suppression of experimental early syphilis by small doses of penicillin comparable to those used in the treatment of gonorrhea. *Am J Syph Gon VD*, 29: 587-596, 1945.
10. Arnold, R. C., Mahoney, J. F. and Cutler, J. C.: Reinfection in experimental syphilis in rabbits following penicillin therapy. I. reinfection in early infectious syphilis. *Am J Syph Gon VD*, 31:264-267, 1947.
11. Arnold, R. C., Mahoney, J. F. and Cutler, J. C.: Reinfection in experimental syphilis in rabbits following penicillin therapy. II. reinfection in early latent syphilis. *Am J Syph Gon VD*, 31:489-492, 1947.
12. Moore, J. E.: *Penicillin in Syphilis*. Springfield, Thomas, 1946.
13. Arnold, R. C., Cutler, J. C., Wright, R. D. and Levitan, S.: Studies in penicillin treatment of syphilis. *Public Health Rep*, 67:78-89, 1952.
14. Hollander, D. H., Turner, T. B. and Nell, E. E.: The effect of long continued subcurative doses of penicillin during the incubation period of experimental syphilis. *Bull Johns Hopkins Hosp*, 90:105-120, 1952.
15. Cutler, J. C., Olansky, S. and Price, E. V.: Treatment of early syphilis: results with penicillin G procaine and two percent aluminum monostearate. *AMA Arch Dermatol*, 71:239-244, 1955.
16. Iskrant, A. P., Bowman, R. W. and Donohue, J. F.: Techniques in evaluation of rapid antisyphilitic therapy. *Public Health Rep*, 63:965-977, 1948.
17. Iskrant, A. P., Remein, Q. R., and Donohue, J. F.: Evaluation of antisyphilitic therapy with intensive follow-up III. statistical method of analysis and its critical evaluation. *J Vener Dis Inform*, 32:371-375, 1951.
18. Plotke, F., Eisenberg, H., Baker, A. H. and Laughlin, M. E.: Penicillin in the Abortive Treatment of Syphilis. A Symposium on Current

Progress in the Study of Venereal Disease, U.S. Government Printing Office, Washington, D.C., 1949, p. 260-266.

19. Alexander, L. J., Schock, A. G. and Mantooth, W. B.: Abortive Treatment of Syphilis. A Symposium on Current Progress in the Study of Venereal Disease, U.S. Government Printing Office, Washington, D.C., 1949, p. 267-271.

20. Woodcock, K. R.: Re-appraising the effect on incubating syphilis of treatment for gonorrhea. *Br J Vener Dis,* 47:95-101, 1971.

CHAPTER 6

FALSE POSITIVE REACTIONS

PART I

NONSYPHILITIC FTA-ABS REACTIONS IN LUPUS ERYTHEMATOSUS

Stephen J. Kraus, M.D.

Two types of serologic tests are available to aid in the diagnosis of syphilis. One type measures antibody against cardiolipin, a substance present in many normal animal tissues. These tests, introduced by Wassermann, are referred to as the nontreponemal tests for syphilis. They differ from one another primarily in the technique for detecting the antibody-cardiolipin reaction such as flocculation (VDRL slide test) or complement fixation (Kolmer test). The nontreponemal test currently used in most laboratories is the VDRL. The second type of serologic tests for syphilis are known as the treponemal tests. They are more specific and utilize as antigen *Treponema pallidum,* the etiologic microorganism of syphilis. Because virulent *T. pallidum* cannot presently be grown *in vitro, T. pallidum* extracted from a rabbit treponemal orchitis is the antigen for these tests. The techniques for measuring the antigen-antibody reaction in the treponemal tests are treponemal immobilization (TPI test), indirect fluorescent antibody (FTA tests), or passive hemagglutination (TPHA).

Wassermann used as antigen for his test an extract of a congenital syphilitic hepar, but shortly thereafter, it was demonstrated that a similar extract of a normal liver gave equivalent results. The fact that normal mammalian tissues and not treponemal antigens were the basis for the cardiolipin tests suggested that reactions in these tests would not be limited to syphilis. Though false positive reactions were diagnosed clinically for many years, the development of the TPI test in 1949 gave laboratory proof to the concept of false positive cardiolipin tests. Studies were then initiated which established the incidence and significance of false positive reactions among various populations (1, 2, 3). For instance, it was found that false positive cardiolipin tests occurred in about 10% of subjects with lupus erythematosus (L.E.) (4, 5) and in certain instances they preceded other serologic tests and clinical signs of L.E. (6, 7, 8).

FTA tests have gone through several stages of development since their initiation by Deacon (9, 10). The FTA 1:5 was the first and although highly sensitive in detecting syphilitic infection, it lacked specificity in that 20-98% of sera from non-syphilitic individuals had a significant reaction in the test (11, 12, 13). The original attempts to reduce these non-syphilis reactions in FTA testing consisted of diluting the sera prior to testing. Several dilutions were advocated but a 1:200 dilution (FTA-200) was chosen as the best compromise between adequate dilution to remove most non-syphilitic reactions and still retain a reaction with a significant number of syphilitic sera (14). The specificity of the FTA-200 test appeared good in normal non-syphilitic subjects, but false positive reactions occurred in certain patients with rheumatoid arthritis (15). These reactions appeared to be related to macroglobulin rheumatoid factor (13). Moreover, the sensitivity of the FTA-200 test did not prove fully adequate.

Further refinement of the FTA tests eventuated in the FTA-ABS test (11). This test's dilution factor is 1:5, but the non-syphilitic reactions of the original FTA 1:5 are blocked by prior incubation of the test sera with sonicate of non-virulent Reiter treponemes or, more recently, by a portion of Reiter liquid culture supernate. The sensitivity of the FTA-ABS was superior to the FTA-200 in detecting syphilis and its high specificity in normals has been documented (11, 12). This high sensitivity and specificity appears to have influenced the interpretation of reactivity sometimes found in sera of patients with disease other than syphilis. Such reactions were thought to indicate syphilis despite the absence of clinical or epidemiologic data supporting this diagnosis (16, 17). Syphilis can coexist with other disease states, but the alternate possibility that a significant number of these reactions could represent false positive FTA-ABS tests was not favored.

The first suggestion of false positive FTA-ABS reactions was that of Macky *et al.* (18) who studied 827 individuals and found 5 cases without a history of syphilis in which the FTA-ABS test was reactive. The fact that these patients had various globulin abnormalities seemed to support the diagnosis of false positive FTA-ABS, yet their old age, the low incidence, and the known sensitivity of the FTA-ABS test made it difficult to absolutely exclude latent or asymptomatic neurosyphilis.

Our investigations on the specificity of the FTA-ABS test were initiated when an atypical pattern of FTA-ABS fluorescence was traced to the sera of three patients with L.E. (19). Instead of the usual homogenous fluorescence of the entire *T. pallidum* antigen, multiple globules, or "beads," of bright fluorescence were scattered along the length of the organism, and the areas between the globules showed little or no fluorescence (Fig. VI-1-A-C). This was termed a beaded pattern of FTA-ABS fluorescence. It must also be differentiated from a pattern seen with an occasional syphilitic serum; one or two bright areas of fluorescence superimposed on homogenous spirochete fluorescence (Fig. VI-1-B). The three patients whose sera produced the beaded fluorescence

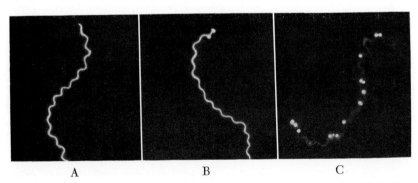

A   B   C

Figure VI-1. Different Fluorescence Patterns Occurring in the FTA-ABS Test. A. Typical homogenous. B. Homogenous with several bright spots. C. Atypical beaded.

had no clinical evidence of syphilis. The fact that this pattern of fluorescence had not been seen with documented syphilitic sera was also against a syphilitic etiology for the atypical fluorescence. However, the small number of observations made it difficult to absolutely exclude concurrent syphilis in these subjects.

An answer to this problem was the objective of a prospective study of FTA-ABS reactions in L.E. (20). This study was designed to further evaluate the possible occurrence of typical homogenous treponeme fluorescence in L.E. and to determine if atypical beaded or typical homogenous fluorescence in L.E. is due to concurrent syphilis. An answer to the latter question was attempted by a thorough search for evidence of prior syphilitic infection and by a statistical comparison of the syphilis serologic tests in the L.E. group with a comparable control group.

One hundred-fifty patients attending a special L.E. clinic at University Hospitals of Cleveland were studied. One hundred-twenty-one had evidence of systemic L.E. and in 29, the disease was limited to cutaneous involvement (discoid L.E.). Control sera were obtained from 75 premarital blood samples drawn at the Fulton County Health Department in Atlanta, Georgia. These samples were chosen prior to testing and individual sera were selected such that the sex and race distribution, and the mean age of the control group matched the L.E. group. In this way the control and L.E. subjects were matched with respect to several variables known to influence the incidence of syphilis. In this way the reactive tests in the control group would represent the expected incidence of reactive tests in the L.E. group based on a syphilitic cause. All sera were tested at the Venereal Disease Research Laboratory and evaluation consisted of the VDRL slide, TPI, and FTA-ABS tests.

Any L.E. or control subject whose serum showed typical or atypical fluorescence in the FTA-ABS test was further evaluated. These patients were questioned for a history of syphilis and were reexamined with special emphasis on evidence of congenital or late syphilis. Cerebrospinal fluid (CSF) examinations were done whenever possible to determine the possibility of asymptomatic neurosyphilis. Total protein, cell count, and VDRL slide tests were performed on the CSF. The syphilis registries in both the city of Cleveland and the state of Ohio were consulted to determine if these patients, their spouses (when married), parents or family members had ever been treated for syphilis or had a reactive serologic test for syphilis.

The results of the serologic testing in both groups are presented in Table 6-I. This table also presents a statistical comparison of results obtained in the L.E. and control groups. Statistically significant differences occurred in the VDRL, atypical beaded FTA-ABS, typical FTA-ABS, and anticomplementary TPI test results. The incidence of these test results was therefore higher in the L.E. group than could be explained by a syphilitic basis. None of the subjects with beaded or homogenous fluorescence in the FTA-ABS was found to have physical findings or a history compatible with prior syphilis infection. The CSF from 7 of these patients was examined and the protein, cells, and VDRL were within normal limits. Syphilis registries in Cleveland and Ohio did not help establish the diagnosis of syphilis in the patients with FTA-ABS fluorescence. The statistical analysis of the data and the results of the clinical and epidemiologic investigations make it extremely unlikely that syphilis could account for the FTA-ABS (typical or atypical), anticomplementary TPI or VDRL reactivities in the L.E. patients. Our observed incidence of false positive VDRL tests was 16% and is consistent with the incidence previously reported in L.E. (4, 5).

TABLE 6-I

COMPARATIVE REACTIVITY OF SEVERAL SEROLOGIC TESTS FOR SYPHILIS IN PATIENTS WITH LUPUS ERYTHEMATOSUS AND IN A CONTROL GROUP OF PATIENTS

Test Results	L.E. Group (150 patients)	Control Group (75 patients)	Degree of Statistical Significance (Chi Square Test)
Reactive VDRL	24*	0	$p < .001$
Atypical FTA-ABS	11	0	$p < .05$
Typical FTA-ABS (borderline and reactive)	12	0	$p < .05$
Anticomplementary TPI	10	0	$p = .05$
Reactive TPI	1	0	Not significant

* Number of patients.

Eight of the 12 sera with homogenous FTA-ABS fluorescence were reported as borderline in reactivity. This supports the current concept that borderline FTA-ABS results are inconclusive for syphilis and should not be interpreted as either reactive or nonreactive (12, 21, 22). The four sera with a reactive FTA-ABS test suggest the factor responsible for homogenous FTA-ABS fluorescence in L.E. may exist in a higher concentration in the sera of certain L.E. patients. The clinician must also realize the reproducibility of the FTA-ABS in the borderline and 1+ reactive range is less than with completely nonreactive specimens or than with 3+ or 4+ reactivity. Thus repetitive testing of a sample initially reported as borderline can occasionally be read as 1+ reactive. Conversely, repetitive testing of a sera initially read as 1+ reactive can occasionally be read as borderline.

The atypical beaded fluorescence was detected by personnel from the Venereal Disease Research Laboratory and the North Carolina State Laboratory. The high intensity of the atypical fluorescence, and the fact that technicians have not been trained to recognize the beaded fluorescence as atypical, raised the question as to what results other laboratories would report with sera producing atypical beaded FTA-ABS reactivity. Such sera samples were therefore sent to two other laboratories and they reported the test results as reactive in the FTA-ABS.

FTA-ABS reactivity in L.E. apparently unrelated to syphilis has subsequently been reported by others (23), yet a previous report on the specificity of the FTA-ABS failed to reveal these reactions (24). The latter study was restricted to individuals with false positive cardiolipin tests for syphilis. The fact that antibodies with different antigenic specificities are involved in the nontreponemal cardiolipin and the treponemal FTA tests suggested to us that sera with false positive cardiolipin reactivity may not necessarily be those that show nonsyphilitic FTA-ABS fluorescence. Although both FTA-ABS fluorescence and cardiolipin reactivity were present in 4 lupus sera, 20 L.E. sera had cardiolipin reactivity without FTA-ABS fluorescence and 19 L.E. sera had FTA-ABS fluorescence without cardiolipin reactivity. Statistical analysis of this data revealed the occurrence of cardiolipin reactivity and FTA-ABS fluorescence in the L.E. group were independent variables (chi square test p $<$ .01). Studies restricted to false positive cardiolipin sera may therefore not have been optimal to detect non-syphilitic FTA-ABS reactivity.

The L.E. serum factors which produce FTA-ABS fluorescence appeared to be globulins and probably antibody, since their detection depended on reaction with fluorescein conjugated anti-human globulin. In further studies (25), IgG, IgA, and IgM specific conjugates were substituted for the usual broad spectrum FTA-ABS conjugate. The antibody responsible for homogenous FTA-ABS fluorescence was restricted primarily to IgG, but the beaded fluorescence was found in all three immunoglobulin classes.

Antibodies with unusual antigen specificities are known to occur in L.E. patients. The possibility that one or more of these antibodies could account for the FTA-ABS reactions in L.E. was evaluated by determining the activity of the sera in the L.E. cell, antinuclear, rheumatoid factor, anti-nucleoprotein, and anti-DNA tests. Similar tests were performed on L.E. sera without FTA-ABS anticity. No statistical correlation was found between homogenous fluorescence and these tests, but beaded FTA-ABS fluorescence was correlated with anti-DNA, anti-nucleoprotein and L.E. cell test activity. This relationship was further established when the beaded FTA-ABS reaction was blocked by prior incubation of the serum with DNA or nucleoprotein, or by prior incubation of the *T. pallidum* antigen with DNAase. These blocking manipulations were without effect on the non-syphilis or syphilis homogenous FTA-ABS reaction.

The relationship of anti-DNA antibodies to beaded FTA-ABS fluorescence has several related implications. Anti-DNA activity correlates with the clinical activity of L.E. and therefore beaded FTA-ABS reactions are more likely to be found with sera from patients with active disease. Such a possibility is supported by the finding of a significant association between beaded FTA-ABS reactions and other correlates of L.E. activity such as the L.E. cell phenomena and nucleoprotein antibodies. Since other disease states can on occasion have anti-DNA activity, beaded FTA-ABS rests might rarely occur in hepatitis, rheumatoid arthritis, glomerulonephritis, scleroderma, and other autoimmune diseases.

The ultrastructure of the beaded FTA-ABS reaction with L.E. sera was studied by substituting a ferritin-anti-human IgG conjugate for the usual fluorescein conjugate (26). This technique demonstrated a similar beaded pattern of L.E. antibody attachment to *T. pallidum*. Antibody attachment could not be localized to treponeme protruding structures, mesosomes, or to particulate rabbit testicular debris. The L.E. antibody did fix to breaks or twists in the outer membrane of *T. pallidum*. This suggests that nuclear material escaped from the treponeme and acted as the antigen in the beaded FTA-ABS reaction.

The finding of non-syphilis reactions in the FTA-ABS test reemphasizes that serologic tests do not themselves diagnose disease but are aids in diagnosis. The physician must be aware of the specificity, sensitivity, and pecularities of a test and then combine the test results with clinical information in establishing a diagnosis. Applying these principles to the FTA-ABS, it can be concluded that this test is the most sensitive of the currently available syphilis serologic tests. Its specificity is good in the general population although even here unexplained reactions occasionally occur (12, 27). Reservations about FTA-ABS specificity must now be made in L.E. and possibly in other disease states having qualitative or quantitative globulin abnormalities. One peculiarity of the FTA-ABS in L.E. is the beaded pattern of fluorescence. If not recognized as atypical in the laboratory, the test results could be reported as reactive, and thus possibly contribute to an erroneous diagnosis of syphilis. On the other hand, awareness of the significance of beaded FTA-ABS fluorescence was the initial clue which aided in the diagnosis of a case of L.E. (28).

SUMMARY

The FTA-ABS test is the most sensitive serologic test for syphilis available today, but its specificity, though high, is not fully defined. Of sera from a group of 150 lupus erythematosus patients, 7.3% gave an atypical, beaded fluorescence pattern when reacted with the *T. pallidum* antigen. Antibodies of the IgG, IgM, and IgA classes participate in the reaction, and they are directed mainly against DNA antigen on the treponeme. An additional 2.6% of the patients gave reactive FTA-ABS results indistinguishable from the typical homogenous staining of the *T. pallidum* sera with syphilis sera, and a further 5.3% of the patients gave typical borderline FTA-ABS test results. A history of syphilis could not be established in any of these patients. These findings remind the physician that serologic tests for syphilis, even though extremely helpful, are only aids in diagnosis, and clinical judgment must be used in their interpretation in unusual circumstances.

REFERENCES

1. Moore, J. E. and Mohr, C. F.: Biologically false positive serologic tests for syphilis type, incidence, and cause. *JAMA* 150:467, 1952.
2. Moore, J. E. and Lutz, W. B.: The natural history of systemic lupus erythematosus: an approach to its study through chronic biologic false positive reactors. *J. Chron. Dis.* 1:297, 1955.
3. Moore, J. E., Shulman, L. E. and Scott, J. T.: The natural history of systemic lupus erythematosus: an approach to its study through chronic biologic false positive reactors. *J. Chron. Dis.* 5:282, 1957.
4. Harvey, A. M., Shulman, L. E., Tumulty, P. A., Conley, C. L. and Schoenrich, E. H.: Systemic lupus erythematosus: review of the literature and clinical analysis of 138 cases. *Medicine* 33:291, 1954.
5. Harvey, A. M. and Shulman, L. E.: In *Lupus Erythematosus* by E. L. Dubois, Chapter 7. New York, McGraw-Hill, 1966.
6. Haserick, J. R. and Long, R.: Systemic lupus erythematosus preceded by false positive serologic tests for syphilis: presentation of five cases. *Ann. Int. Med.* 37:559, 1952.
7. Knight, A. and Wilkinson, R. D.: The clinical significance of the biological false positive serologic reactor: a study of 113 cases. *Canad. Med. Ass. J.* 88:1193, 1963.
8. Putkonen, T., Jokinen, E. J., Lassus, A. *et al.*: Chronic biologic false positive seroreactions for syphilis as a harbinger of systemic lupus erythematosus. *Acta. Derm.* 47:83, 1967.
9. Deacon, W. E., Freeman, Elizabeth M. and Harris, A.: Fluorescent treponemal antibody test. Modification based on quantitation (FTA-200). *Proc. Soc. Exp. Biol. Med.* 103:827, 1960.
10. Deacon, W. E. and Freeman, E. M.: Fluorescent treponemal antibody studies. *J. Invest. Derm.* 34:249, 1960.

11. Hunter, E. F., Deacon, W. E. and Meyer, P. E.: An improved FTA test for syphilis: The absorption procedure (FTA-ABS). *Pub. Health Rep.* 79:410, 1964.

12. Goldman, J. N. and Lantz, M. A.: FTA-ABS and VDRL slide test reactivity: in a population of nuns. *JAMA* 217:53, 1971.

13. Wilkinson, A. E. and Rayner, C. F. A.: Studies on the fluorescent treponemal antibody (FTA) test. *Brit. J. Vener. Dis.* 42:8, 1966.

14. Deacon, W. E., Freeman, E. M. and Harris, A.: Fluorescent treponemal antibody test. Modification based on quantitation (FTA-200). *Proc. Soc. Exp. Biol. Med.* 103:827, 1960.

15. Fife, E. H.: *Proc. World Forum on Syphilis and Other Treponematoses*, p. 254, U.S.P.H.S. publication No. 997, Washington, D. C., 1962.

16. Wood, R. M., Yoshihiko, I., Argonza, W., Bradford, L., Jue, R., Jeong, Y., Puffer, J. and Bodily, H. L.: Comparison of the fluorescent treponemal antibody absorption and *treponemal pallidum* immobilization tests on serums from 1182 diagnostic problem cases. *Am. J. Clin. Path.* 47:521, 1967.

17. Deacon, W. E., Lucas, J. B. and Price, E. V.: Fluorescent treponemal antibody-absorption (FTA-ABS) test for syphilis. *JAMA* 198:624, 1966.

18. Mackey, D. M., Price, E. V., Knox, J. M. and Scotti, A.: Specificity of the FTA-ABS test for syphilis: an evaluation. *JAMA* 207:1683, 1969.

19. Kraus, S. J., Haserick, J. R. and Lantz, M. A.: Atypical FTA-ABS test fluorescence in lupus erythematous patients. *JAMA* 211:2140, 1970.

20. Kraus, S. J., Haserick, J. R. and Lantz, M. A.: Fluorescent treponemal antibody-absorption test reactions in lupus erythematosus. *New Eng. J. Med.* 282:1287, 1970.

21. Cohen, P., Stout, G. and Ende, N.: Serologic reactivity in consecutive patients admitted to a general hospital. A comparison of the FTA-ABS, VDRL and automated reagin tests. *Arch. Intern. Med.* 124:364, 1969.

22. *Manual of Tests for Syphilis*, Public Health Service Publication 411. U.S. Dept. of Health, Education, and Welfare, Government Printing Office, 1969.

23. Jokinen, E. J., Lassus, A. and Linder, E.: Fluorescent treponemal antibody reaction in sera with antinuclear factors. *Ann. Clin. Res.* 1:77, 1969.

24. Wuepper, K. D., Bodily, H. L. and Tuffanelli, D. L.: Serologic tests for syphilis and the false-positive reactor. *Arch. Derm.* 94:152, 1966.

25. Kraus, S. J., Haserick, J. R., Logan, L. C. and Bullard, J. C.: Atypical fluorescence in the fluorescent treponemal-antibody-absorption (FTA-ABS) test related to deoxyribonucleic acid (DNA) antibodies. *J. Immunol.* 106:1665, 1971.

26. Strobel, P. L. and Kraus, S. J.: An electron microscopic study of the FTA-ABS "beading" phenomenon with lupus erythematosus sera, using ferritin-conjugated anti-human IgG. *J. Immunol.* 108:1152, 1972.

27. Buchanan, C. S. and Haserick, J. R.: FTA-ABS test in pregnancy. A probable false-positive reaction. *Arch. Derm.* 102:322, 1970.

28. Kraus, S. J. and Daniels, K. C.: Atypical FTA-ABS test reaction. *Arch. Derm.* (in press).

PART II

NORMAL INDIVIDUALS WITH CHRONIC FALSE POSITIVE (CFP) TESTS FOR SYPHILIS

Denny L. Tuffanelli

INTRODUCTION

THE CLINICAL MANAGEMENT of patients with chronic false positive (CFP) serologic tests for syphilis is complicated by the fact that the prognostic implication of CFP serology is incompletely understood.

Wassermann antibody may be a means of recognizing individuals with a basic abnormality of immune response long before they develop tissue damage (10). It is found in 20 percent of patients with systemic lupus erythematosus (SLE) (9). Cases have been presented in which false positive reactions have antedated the development of frank SLE by many years (16, 20). In general, however, these cases were highly selected and usually were initially seen because of clinical symptoms of a connective tissue disorder.

The purpose of the present study was to determine the incidence of development of systemic disease, particularly SLE, in patients who present initially CFP serological reactions for syphilis. In a long-term survey of CFP reactors the clinical and laboratory findings in 49 normal individuals with false positive VDRL tests followed for two to eight years are reported.

STUDY GROUPS AND METHODS

The study group consists of 142 CFP reactors who have been followed over the last eight years at the Department of Dermatology, University of California Medical Center, San Francisco. The mode of presentation in these patients was mixed. Initial serologies were done in the following situations: pregnancy, VD clinic and hospital investigation of a systemic disease. In addi-

95

tion, a large number of patients were seen initially in a referral clinic for patients with connective tissue disorders. Over 700 false positive reactors, transient and chronic, have been studied to date. The CFP reactors were seen at one to six month intervals in most instances. All have had at least 4 and sometimes as many as 15 separate specimens of serum taken at intervals. Criteria for diagnosis of CFP serological test for syphilis include a repeatedly positive VDRL and negative TPI and FTA-ABS tests (15). CFP reactors had repeatedly positive reagin tests, persisting longer than six months. Because of the possibility of aging per se being a cause for CFP reactions, data on 20 healthy CFP reactors over age 60 followed in our clinic were not included in this study. Blood was drawn by venipuncture for the following studies: venereal disease research laboratory tests (VDRL), *treponema pallidum* immobilization test (TPI), fluorescent treponemal antibody absorption test (FTA-ABS), LE-cell preparation, latex fixation for rheumatoid factor and antinuclear antibody determination (ANA). Serum IgG, IgA and IgM levels were measured quantitatively.

Sixty of the CFP patients had underlying systemic disease, 33 were drug addicts and 49 had no clinical disease. This report will deal primarily with the 49 healthy patients.

RESULTS

The clinical diagnoses of the 142 patients with CFP serologies are listed in Table 6-II. Sixty of the patients had diseases usually classified as *autoimmune,* and the most common diagnosis was systemic lupus erythematosus (35 patients). Four patients had discoid lupus erythematosus, with the only serologic abnormality being a positive serology. All 60 of these patients were seen initially by us because of systemic disease and were found when examined to have CFP serologies. Eight gave a history of false positive serologies prior to the present diagnosis. In 6 of the 8, however, signs or symptoms of their disease probably existed before the serologies became positive. Thirty-nine of 310 (7.9 percent) patients with lupus erythematosus studied had CFP serologies.

TABLE 6-II

CFP REACTORS FOR SYPHILIS

Clinical Diagnosis	No. of Patients
Lupus erythematosus	35
Discoid lupus	4
Rheumatoid arthritis	6
Idiopathic thrombocytopenic purpura	2
Malignancy	3
Scleroderma	2
Hemolytic anemia	2
Thyroiditis	2
Ulcerative colitis	1
Erythema nodosum	1
Vasculitis	1
Atopic dermatitis	1
Narcotic addiction	33
No disease	49
Total	142

Thirty-three of the patients were narcotic addicts. Serological and clinical studies of the narcotic addicts (22) and patients with systemic disease (20) have been previously reported by us.

Forty-nine of the patients were *healthy* at the time of this study. These patients were seen initially, in most instances, in a VD clinic or during pregnancy. In this group forty-one were females and eight were males. The average age when seen by us was 24, with a range of 13 to 60. The patients were followed at three to six months intervals, when possible, for two to eight years with the average time of observation 4.9 years.

In eight of these patients the VDRL titer obtained was higher than eight dilutions; in most it was positive at two to four dils. High titer false positive reactions have been noted and have been previously reported (24). Sera changed in titer from time to time and were negative for varying periods of time in individual patients.

Table 6-IV records the incidence of serological abnormalities in the three categories of CFP reactors: Those with systemic disease, narcotic addicts and *healthy* patients. While numerous abnormalities are noted in the group with systemic disease, no major abnormalities are noted in those patients who presented ini-

TABLE 6-III

VDRL TITER IN "HEALTHY" CFP REACTORS

Highest titer obtained is recorded.

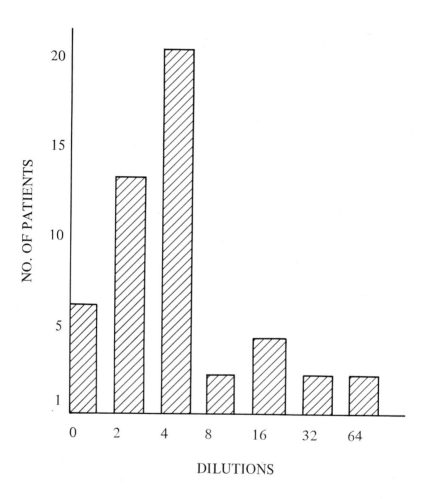

TABLE 6-IV

INCIDENCE OF SEROLOGIC ABNORMALITIES IN CFP* REACTORS

	Systemic Disease			Drug Addicts			"Healthy"		
	No.	Posi-tive	Per-cent	No.	Posi-tive	Per-cent	No.	Posi-tive	Per-cent
HGG†	60	25	41.6	33	10	30.3	49	9	10.3
ANA	60	40	66.6	33	4	12.1	49	6	12.2
RF‡	60	18	30.0	33	4	12.1	49	5	10.2
LE factor	60	28	44.2	33	0	0	49	0	0

* CFP indicates chronic false positive.
† HGG indicated hypergammaglobulinemia.
‡ RF indicates rheumatoid factor.

tially CFP serologies and remained healthy during the period of observation.

Quantitative immunoglobulin levels are listed in Table 6-IV. The only abnormality noted was the elevation of IgM in CFP reactors with systemic disease ($P = 0.03$).

During the period of time they were followed in our clinic, none of the *healthy* CFP reactors developed signs or symptoms of systemic disease. All were asymptomatic at the time of last examination.

DISCUSSION

Despite intensive study since their acceptance as authoritative tests for syphilis, the various serological examinations for syphilis have many confusing aspects. Positive tests have been associated with a variety of diseases, and an increased incidence has been observed in the elderly.

The frequency of positive serological reactions for syphilis varies greatly with composition of the series and the sensitivity

TABLE 6-V

IMMUNOGLOBULIN LEVELS IN CFP REACTORS AND NORMALS

	No. Subjects Studied	IgG (mg/100 cu)	IgA (mg/100 cu)	IgM (mg/100 cu)
CFP with systemic disease ...	60	1230 ± 270	174 ± 52	142 ± 71
CFP "healthy"	49	1205 ± 330	141 ± 78	106 ± 38
Normals	66	1150 ± 214	168 ± 52	105 ± 54

of the serological tests employed. In the present series only the VDRL test was used as a screening procedure. One hundred forty-two CFP reactors have been obtained from a much larger number of false positive reactors and followed in a long-term clinical and serological survey. All were characterized by the continuous or intermittent production of reagin.

Reagin (Wassermann antibody) is a ubiquitous serum protein that may indicate syphilis or occasional predisposition to a disease of immunologic aberration. Patients with serum reagin and nonreactive treponemal-antibody tests have classically been considered to have *biologic* false-positive seroreactions.

The various disorders associated with false positive reactions have been extensively documented. Acute or transient reactions are associated with viral, bacterial, plasmodial and spirochetal infections, smallpox vaccinations (7) and pregnancy (17).

Chronic false positive reactions are associated with lupus erythematosus, Hashimoto's thyroiditis and other diseases of immunologic aberration (18, 20). Lepromatous leprosy (14, 19) and brucellosis are the major infectious diseases involved. Aging (1, 21) and narcotic addiction (3, 8, 22) are interesting and poorly understood causes. An increased incidence in professional blood donors has recently been reported (5).

In Harvey's (9, 10) series of 192 CFP reactors, 29 percent had systemic illness; 43 percent were healthy but had evidence of a serum protein abnormality and in 28 percent there was no evidence of serologic or clinical abnormality. Serological abnormalities suggesting autoimmune disease have been frequently reported in CFP reactors. Doniach and others (4) reported 51 CFP reactors in whom 46 percent had antinuclear antibodies, 24 percent had smooth muscle antibodies and 51 percent had mitochondrial antibodies. The series is somewhat weighted in that over half the patients were general hospital cases investigated for systemic disease.

Relatives of CFP reactors have also been shown to have an increased incidence of antinuclear antibodies, hypergammaglobulin and elevated IgM levels (23). No increased incidence of clinical disease was noted in the relatives. However, such series are usually weighted by the fact that the patients are usually gathered in part at least from general hospital cases, collagen disease clinics, etc.

Our own data concerning the *incidence* of systemic disease in CFP reactors is biased by the fact that many of the patients were seen initially in a collagen disease clinic. Eight percent of our patients with SLE had CFP serologies, and inclusion of these patients obviously gives a biased sample. Thus we would make no conclusion concerning the incidence of disease in our CFP reactors. This also tends to confuse the integration of data. The possibility of false positive FTA-ABS is, of course, present and tends to complicate the problem further.

Goldman and Lantz (6) studied 250 celibate nuns. Of these, only 2 (1 percent) probably had false positive FTA-ABS. The cause in these patients was unknown. Jacobs and others (11) have reported an apparent transient false positive FTA-ABS test following smallpox vaccination. Mackey and others (13) reported five patients of 827 tested who had reactive FTA-ABS, nonreactive TPI tests and no clinical or historical evidence to suggest syphilis. This incidence represents 0.6 percent of the total tested.

The results of the FTA-ABS test in lupus erythematosus can be particularly confusing. Kraus and others (12) studied 150 patients with SLE. The VDRL test was reactive in twenty-four. Twenty-three patients showed some degree of fluorescence in the FTA-ABS test; of these, four were reactive (one had a positive TPI) and eight were borderline. In the other eleven, an atypical *beading* fluorescence pattern was noted. VDRL reactivity and FTA-ABS fluorescence are independent variables with no apparent link (6).

The prognosis of patients with CFP reactors has always been implied to be poor. Harvey (9, 10) reported a study of 192 chronic CFP reactors discovered mainly at examination for a health certificate at prenatal clinics and at medical examination for military service. In two of 192 subjects the primary examination also revealed SLE. During the observation period ranging from two to twenty-five years (average twelve years), Hashimoto's thyroditis developed in three and SLE in a further twelve. Berglund and Carlsson (2) studied thirty-nine chronic

CFP reactors. One had SLE at the beginning of the observation period. During the observation period, SLE developed in one woman and probable SLE in another. Nine of twenty-two studied had ANA.

Putkonen (16) has studied the same problem. Eighty-one chronic false positive reactors were followed. The mean follow-up time was five years. The group was primarily gathered from hospital patients. In four, SLE was present before antilipoidal tests for syphilis turned reactive. In thirteen patients definite or probable SLE developed within two years, and in one case 4.5 years after the detection of the CFP phenomenon. In six patients chronic SLE ensued eight to twenty-three years after the discovery of the false positive seroreactions.

The probability of developing a definite SLE in this series was 6 percent for the sixteen men and 22 percent for the sixty-five women. It was 60 percent for the ten girls who were twenty years of age or younger when the false positive seroreactions were detected. The authors concluded that in men the CFP phenomenon rarely heralds SLE, but in women it is a more ominous sign. Especially in young women a subacute to fulminant type of SLE was thought to develop concurrently or within two years after detection of the false positive seroreactions.

Salo and others (17) are studying a more valid CFP group in attempting to answer the question of prognosis. From 141,043 sera from pregnant women, twenty-eight chronic CFP reactors have been obtained. Follow-up studies are being performed but have not been reported (17).

Our data do not substantiate the concept that a CFP serology implies a serious prognosis. None of the forty-nine patients developed systemic disease during the period of observation. In particular, seven girls initially studied under the age of twenty-one remain perfectly healthy.

During the observation period, which was on the average 4.9 years, no patients developed signs or symptoms of systemic disease. From these studies one can also conclude that Wassermann reagin is not, in itself, harmful to the individual.

Our data would indicate that the presence of a CFP serology in the absence of signs or symptoms of systemic disease is not necessarily a serious prognostic sign. Patients with this finding should not be unduly alarmed. Serologic and clinical studies of the presence of systemic disease should, however, be performed.

REFERENCES

Aho, K.: Studies of syphilitic antibodies. 3. Anamnestic reactions and 19 S predominance of the anti-lipoidal antibodies in aged persons. *Br J Vener Dis,* 44:283, 1968.

Berglund, S. and Carlsson, M.: Clinical significance of chronic biologic false positive Wassermann reaction and "antinuclear factors." *Acta Med Scand,* 180:407, 1966.

Cherubin, C. E. and Millian, S. J.: Serologic investigations in narcotic addicts. I. Syphilis, lymphogranuloma venereum, herpes simplex and Q fever. *Ann Intern Med,* 69:739, 1968.

Doniach, D., Delhanty, J., Lindqvist, H. J. and Catterall, R. D.: Mitochondrial and other tissue autoantibodies in patients with biological false positive reactions for syphilis. *Clin Exp Immunol,* 6:871, 1970.

Garner, M. F.: The biological false positive reaction to serologic tests for syphilis. *J Clin Pathol,* 23:31, 1970.

Goldman, J. N. and Lantz, M. A.: FTA-ABS and VDRL slide test reactivity in a population of nuns. *JAMA,* 217:53, 1971.

Grossman, L. J. and Peery, T. M.: Biologically false positive serologic tests for syphilis due to smallpox vaccination. *Am J Clin Pathol,* 51:375, 1969.

Harris, W. D. M. and Andrei, J.: Serologic tests for syphilis among narcotic addicts. *NY State J Med,* 2967, 1967.

Harvey, A. M.: Auto-immune disease and the chronic biologic false positive test for syphilis. *JAMA,* 182:513, 1962.

Harvey, A. M. and Shulman, L. E.: Connective tissue disease and the chronic biologic false positive test for syphilis (BFP reaction). *Med Clin North Am,* 50:1271, 1966.

Jacobs, M. J., Prothro, G. W. and Carpenter, R. L.: Apparent transient false positive FTA-ABS test following smallpox vaccination. *Morbidity and Mortality Weekly Report,* Jan. 30, 1971.

Kraus, S. J., Haserick, J. R. and Lantz, M. A.: Fluorescent treponemal antibody absorption test reactions in lupus erythematosus. *N Engl J Med,* 282:1287, 1970.

Mackey, D. M., Price, E. V., Knox, J. M. and Scotti, A.: Specificity of the FTA-ABS test for syphilis. *JAMA,* 207:1683, 1969.

Matthews, L. J. and Trautman, J. R.: Clinical and serological profiles in leprosy. *Lancet:* 915, 1965.

Nicholas, L.: Serodiagnosis of syphilis. *Arch Dermatol,* 96:324, 1967.

Putkonen, T., Jokinen, E. J., Lassus, A. and Mustakallio, K. K.: Chronic biologic false positive seroreactions for syphilis as a harbinger of systemic lupus erythematosus. *Acta Derm Venereol,* 47:83, 1967.

Salo, O. P., Aho, K., Nieminen, E. and Hormila, P.: False positive serological test for syphilis in pregnancy. *Acta Derm Venereol*, 49:332, 1969.

Salo, O. P., Sievers, K., Ahvonen, P. and Aho, K.: Low frequency of chronic biological false positive reactors to serologic tests for syphilis in rheumatoid arthritis and ankylosing spondylitis. *Ann Rheum Dis*, 27:261, 1968.

Scotti, A. T., Mackey, D. M. and Trautman, J. R.: Syphilis and biologic false positive reactors among leprosy patients. *Arch Dermatol*, 101:328, 1970.

Tuffanelli, D. L., Wuepper, K. D., Bradford, L. L. and Wook, R. M.: Fluorescent treponemal antibody absorption tests. Studies of false positive reactions to tests for syphilis. *N Engl J Med*, 276:265, 1967.

Tuffanelli, D. L.: Ageing and false positive reactions for syphilis. *Br J Vener Dis*, 42:40, 1967.

Tuffanelli, D. L.: Narcotic addiction with false positive reaction for syphilis. Immunologic studies. *Acta Derm Venereol*, 48:542, 1968.

Tuffanelli, D. L.: False positive reactions for syphilis. Serologic abnormalities in relatives of chronic reactors. *Arch Dermatol*, 98:606, 1968.

Wuepper, K. D. and Tuffanelli, D. L.: False positive reaction to VDRL test with prozone phenomena. Association with lymphosarcoma. *JAMA*, 195:868, 1966.

CHAPTER 7

VENEREAL DISEASE IN THE MILITARY

With Special Reference to Incidence and Management in Southeast Asia

COMMANDER THOMAS E. CARSON

AND

DAVID W. JOHNSON

INCIDENCE*

VENEREAL DISEASE incidence remains a primary concern of military commanders since combat effectiveness can be directly limited if large numbers of personnel are involved. Loss of man hours, transportation tie-ups and facilities required for care are of significance when units report annual case rates of over 50/1000 strength. Some units in Southeast Asia have reported case rates in excess of 500/1000!

During major conflicts in the past, case rates actually fell during the campaigns but increased in the demobilization periods. Table 7-I illustrates a decline in case rates after the post World War II rise. This was probably due in part to the penicillin panacea and resultant laxity in reporting. After the Korean War ending in 1953, there was a relatively gentle increase followed by a later decline.

---

* Statistical data in this section is primarily from Navy-Marine Corps material. Continental United States figures correlate well with other military services while outside United States figures primarily indicate Pacific Theater case rates.

A different trend in case rates has occurred in the Vietnamese conflict. Table 7-II shows a definite and steady rise in annual case rates among U.S. military men outside the continental U.S. which parallels the general worldwide increase in venereal disease for all the population during 1966 to 1970. The alarming increase occurred in the Vietnam theater. This rise during the

TABLE 7-I

U.S. NAVY AND MARINE CORPS COMBINED SYPHILIS AND
GONORRHEA INCIDENCE RATES PER 1,000 AVERAGE ANNUAL
STRENGTH—FISCAL YEARS 1947 THROUGH 1964

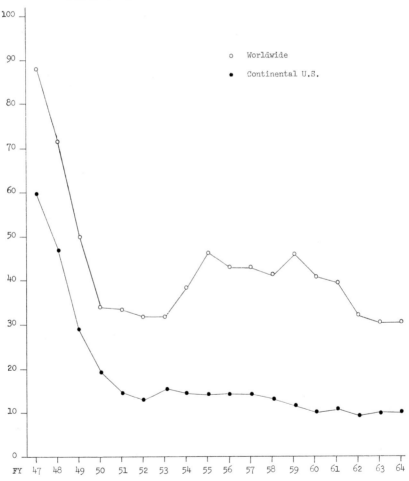

TABLE 7-II

U.S. NAVY AND MARINE CORPS COMBINED VENEREAL DISEASE
INCIDENCE RATE PER 1,000 AVERAGE ANNUAL STRENGTH
FISCAL YEAR 1966 THROUGH 1970

Fiscal Year	Continental U.S.	Outside Continental U.S.*	Vietnam Only
1966	9.4	48.3	39.2
1967	19.0	68.6	112.9
1968	20.7	68.6	107.5
1969	21.6	70.6	90.9
1970	24.2	86.8	183.1

* Includes Vietnam, all ships and all stations outside the Continental United States.

major part of the war from 1967 to 1970 is a reflection that the Vietnamese campaign was different from other wars in which the United States has been involved. We were in more of an advisory capacity with more personnel involved in logistical support and there were more regularly scheduled leaves to such places as Taiwan, Hong Kong, Thailand and Japan.

FACTORS INFLUENCING CASE RATES

Among the factors having a direct or indirect bearing on case rates is the energy applied to the reporting system. Preventive medicine units responsible for reporting infectious disease were sparse in the northernmost section of South Vietnam in 1966. By 1967 when venereal disease became recognized as a significant infectious disease problem, more venereal disease control personnel were assigned to preventive medicine units, and as seen in Table 7-II, there was a sharp rise in the incidence of venereal disease. The rise was partially due to an improved reporting system.

Table 7-III demonstrates that venereal disease case rates vary tremendously in a military population according to geographic location. It can be seen that the chancroid case rate in Navy-Marine Corps personnel in Vietnam was over forty times that in personnel stationed in the continental United States.

Another important factor is the age range of the population

TABLE 7-III

INCIDENCE OF VENEREAL DISEASE BY TYPE AND GEOGRAPHIC
LOCATION—U.S. NAVY AND MARINE CORPS FISCAL YEAR 1970

Diagnosis	Continental U.S.		Outside U.S.		Vietnam	
	Number	Rate per 1,000	Number	Rate per 1,000	Number	Rate per 1,000
Total	11,754	24.2	42,169	78.1	13,347	183.1
Syphilis	333	0.7	781	1.4	103	1.4
Gonorrhea	11,296	23.3	40,109	74.3	12,624	173.2
Chancroid	125	0.2	1,279	2.4	620	8.5

being studied. The Navy-Marine Corps gonorrhea case rate in
the continental United States, fiscal year 1970, was 23.3 per 1000
average strength as compared to only 2.9 per 1000 in the general
civilian population. A more appropriate comparison, however,
is with the civilian rate for males between the ages of 20 to 24
which was 25.4 per 1000 for fiscal year 1970 and exceeds the rate
in Navy-Marine Corps personnel stationed in the continental
United States. This emphasizes the fact that military venereal
disease case rates, although high, apply primarily to young adult,
sexually active males.

Venereal disease rates are highest in the military overseas.
There are a number of superficially apparent reasons which include the availability of prostitutes, loneliness, boredom and the
termination of parental control. Tales of exploits are common
in groups of men living together in close quarters, and a young
man is encouraged to prove his manhood. There is a need to go
along with whatever others are doing. Combat situations stimulate *here today, gone tomorrow* attitudes and despite *off limits*
warnings, men will knowingly take extra, punishable risks to find
female contacts. Prostitution flourishes near many military in-
stallations overseas, and venereal disease incidence is highest
when there is little or no control effort by foreign civil authorities.

CONTROL MEASURES

Historically, almost every conceivable venereal disease control
measure has been tried, and as is evident from statistical material, none has been very successful. Harsh punishment of prosti-

tutes (as practiced in some areas of South Vietnam) has not been effective. Punishment of patients with venereal disease resulted in failure of infected personnel to seek treatment and a subsequent increase in complications. Placing responsibility for maintaining low venereal disease case rates on unit commanders as a measure of their leadership led to falsified reports and reluctance of subordinates to seek treatment for fear of punishment.

The use of prophylactic ointments, intraurethral irrigations and mandatory cleansing at prophylactic stations had limited success and have been discontinued. Low dosage prophylactic antibiotics are no longer recommended because of possible sensitization. The low dosages used would appear to contribute to development of resistant strains of bacteria.

Licensing and periodic examination of prostitutes in areas surrounding military camps has been difficult to sustain, and the concerns of our society has limited its use. This is an area for consideration, however, because Japan, where licensing of prostitutes was practiced for a period, became one of the more *low incidence* areas in the Orient.

The primary control measure used by the military today is education in disease prevention. Films, posters and *handouts* are available to medical officers for use in training. Past experience indicates that a lowered venereal disease incidence rate can be achieved by holding periodic informal discussions with small groups of men, systematically covering the entire unit. The lay military is interested in this subject, and many questions will be brought out which tend to eliminate misinformation so common in stories about venereal disease. The proper use of condoms, early recognition of disease and necessity for prompt treatment are easily discussed. It can be explained that the medical restriction which confines patients to their station or ship during treatment is necessary to prevent spread of disease rather than a form of punishment.

Punishment of any form for reporting for treatment of venereal disease is prohibited in the military; however, a person with repeated venereal infections can be separated from the service for behavioral maladjustment.

ASPECTS OF VENERAL DISEASE MANAGEMENT
PECULIAR TO THE MILITARY

Uncontrolled prostitution, most commonly encountered outside the U.S., results in an increase in venereal disease, and the priority for providing treatment detracts from prevention effort. A significant percentage of clinical effort is devoted to these problems. Over 15 percent of Navy and Marine dermatology outpatients seen in Da Nang, Vietnam during 1967 were referred for diagnosis and treatment of diseases of the genitalia (Table 7-IV). Only one-half were true venereal disease; however, other conditions such as pyogenic penile ulcers, so common in a tropical environment, require as much diagnostic work-up as chancroid and syphilis.

Another problem encountered, especially in a combat area, is transportation of patients. It is necessary to keep medical evacuation transports (helicopters, planes, boats, trucks and occasionally tanks) available for movement of injured and more severely ill patients. Venereal disease treatment must often be delayed and when treated, patients must be immediately returned to their primary duty to maintain their unit's combat effectiveness. Follow-up is frequently impossible.

TABLE 7-IV

PERCENTAGE OF VENEREAL AND NONVENEREAL DISEASES
OF THE GENITALIA

	Percent
1. Gonorrhea	2.8
2. Balanitis	2.7
3. Pyogenic Penile Ulcers	2.5
4. Condyloma Acuminatum	2.5
5. Chancroid	2.0
6. Nonspecific Urethritis	1.5
7. Syphilis	.7
8. Herpes Progenitalis	.5
9. Lymphogranuloma	.4
10. Prostatitis	.4
11. Pediculosis	.1
12. Scabies	.1
Total	16.2

(Analysis of over 13,500 dermatology outpatients, Da Nang, RVN, 1967.)

Setting up and keeping facilities with staining methods, serology, dark-field microscopy and culture materials is at times difficult. Especially troublesome is on the job training of new paramedical personnel in the special techniques required for adequate diagnosis of venereal disease. Inherent in the military is the periodic rotation of trained technicians.

There are certain advantages in dealing with venereal disease in the military. The large volume of venereal disease justifies assigning preventive medicine, paramedical and medical personnel to the problem with resultant expertise in case finding, diagnosis and management. Special centers for diagnosis and research can be established. There is an element of control over the patient in a military organization. Health records go with the military man from duty station to duty station aiding good follow-up practices, and although problematical, persons on active duty can be located and follow-up information retrieved.

Uniformity in medical management is encouraged by military headquarters who can consult with recognized authorities and distribute new information and recommendations to all units on a regular basis.

DIAGNOSTIC METHODS

The purpose of this discussion is to outline a simplified diagnostic approach to venereal and nonvenereal diseases of the genitalia. This approach has been found to be adequate to handle most of the venereal disease problem even where limited facilities restrict more sophisticated methods of study. More detail is presented under specific disease headings.

Stains

Gram's stain of the material from all urethral discharges and genital lesions is an essential step for diagnosis. This should be obtained by touching the glass slide to a drop of pus from the urethra or to the unaltered genital lesion. In this way, formations of bacteria (important in the diagnosis of chancroid) will not be disrupted.

As will be outlined later, Wright's or Geimsa's stain may be necessary for the rare diagnosis of granuloma inguinale and confirmation of suspected herpes progenitalis.

Frei Test

Skin testing with Frei antigen (available commercially) is the simplest method for excluding lymphopathia venereum. This test is usually positive within two to five weeks after the appearance of clinical lymphadenopathy. Both antigen and control are placed intradermally and the sites inspected in forty-eight to seventy-two hours. A positive is reported when induration of at least six millimeters is palpable at the antigen injection site and the control is negative. Skin reactivity persists for many years and may merely indicate past infection.

Serologic Tests for Syphilis (STS)

Adequate serological testing is essential in the detection and follow-up of syphilis. One reliable flocculation test such as the Venereal Disease Research Laboratory (VDRL) test with dilution titers should be available. Of course, the Fluorescent Treponemal Antibody absorbed (FTA-ABS) test is invaluable in differentiating a biologic false positive reaction from syphilis (discussed in another chapter) but for the usual screening of large numbers of patients and follow-up of treated disease, a flocculation test is all that is absolutely necessary.

Where facilities for controlled flocculation studies are lacking, the Rapid Plasma Reagin (RPR) test may be used for screening and gross titers can be obtained by diluting the serum.

Dark-field Microscopy

If possible, a specimen should be taken from all genital lesions for dark-field microscopy.* Lesions of early syphilis may be masked by secondary infection or occur in conjunction with one or more of the other venereal diseases and cannot therefore be diagnosed by clinical inspection alone.

After material for Gram's stain is taken, the lesion should be soaked and gently cleansed with saline for twenty to thirty minutes to remove all excess purulent material and debris. The lesion is touched with a clean slide to obtain a small amount of

---

* Any spirocheticidal drug recently administered to the patient negates the value of dark-field microscopy.

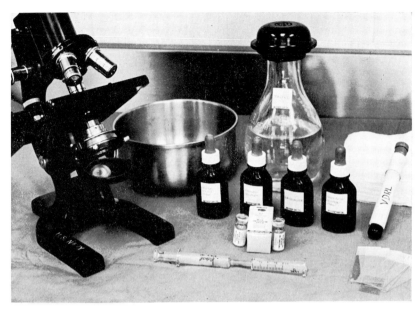

Figure VII-1. Materials necessary for venereal disease diagnosis.

exudate. This step can be facilitated by applying negative pressure to the cleansed lesion with the syringe apparatus shown in Figure VII-1. It can be constructed by removing the plunger from a 2 ml syringe and joining this at the small end with a short rubber tube to a 2 or 5 ml syringe. The mouth of the open syringe is then placed over the lesion and negative pressure applied by pulling on the plunger of the second syringe.

One or two drops of saline are mixed with the exudate on the slide and then examined under a coverslip edged with petrolatum to prevent drying. A microscope equipped with a dark-field adapter and an oil immersion objective is used. *Treponema pallidum* appears as a birefringent slender rod with six to twelve coils (Fig. VII-2) and moves along its long axis in a slow, deliberate fashion. One morphologically sound organism is enough for a positive report.

Material for dark-field microscopy may be aspirated from suspicious lymph nodes by first introducing .2 to .3 ml of sterile saline into the center of the node through an 18-gauge needle.

The entire field under the coverslip should be scanned syste-

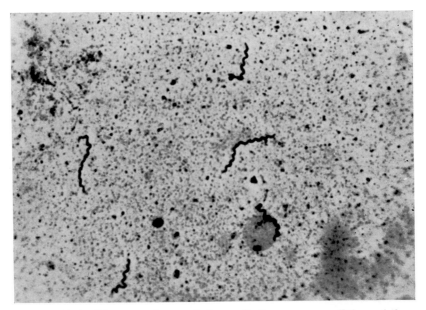

Figure VII-2. The typical morphology of *Treponema pallidum* (silver stain × 930).

matically. This usually requires twenty to thirty minutes by a skilled technician. Falsely negative findings are all too frequent, and clinically suspicious lesions should be reexamined two or three times at twenty-four-hour intervals before any treatment is initiated.

Cultures

Culture facilities are not absolutely necessary for managing venereal disease in males but are useful in treatment failures, determining antibiotic sensitivities and periodic correlation with the reading of Gram's stains. Ideally, unaltered exudate from the urethra or genital lesion should be taken with a wire loop and directly plated on selective media. Media for venereal disease diagnosis should include blood agar, chocolate agar and Thayer-Martin. The blood agar plates should be incubated aerobically, and the chocolate agar and Thayer-Martin medium placed under increased CO_2 tension.

Some organisms are extremely susceptible to desiccation, and therefore falsely negative cultures may be obtained if not directly inoculated from the lesion as outlined above. For gonococci, a commercially available modification of Thayer-Martin medium (Transgrow) may have value for clinics with limited facilities.

In summary, basic requirements for operating an adequate venereal disease clinic include facilities for Gram's stains, lymphopathia venereum skin tests, serologic tests for syphilis and dark-field microscopy.

GONORRHEA

Gonorrhea remains the most prevalent venereal disease in the military in spite of relatively rapid, simple and effective techniques for diagnosis and therapy. This indicates a problem in control of infected persons and detection of asymptomatic carriers. Case rates in military units are related to access of personnel to the surrounding civilian population. Limiting spread of the disease is dependent upon sound public health measures of adequate reporting, investigation of contacts, prompt effective treatment and health education.

Man is the only reservoir, and infection is acquired through direct, intimate contact of a susceptible individual with an infected host. The organism is unable to penetrate normal skin, hence mucous membranes are the usual portal of entry.

Diagnosis

The causative organism, *Neisseria gonorrhoeae* is a gram-negative kidney bean shaped diplococcus. The incubation period is relatively constant with the onset of symptoms between three and six days following exposure. The predominate symptom is a burning sensation during urination inside the urethral canal at the glans, followed by a profuse thick purulent yellow-white urethral discharge. The most common complications involve the prostate, seminal vesicles and epididymis. Pelvic pain and tenderness and fever accompany their enlargement.

Rarely, septicemia, arthritis and metastatic skin lesions may complicate gonococcal urethritis. Metastatic lesions are characterized by hemorrhagic, crusted vesiculopustules chiefly occurring on the hands and feet.

Cutaneous gonorrhea (Fig. VII-3) or gonococcal pyoderma is not uncommon in a tropical environment. This condition is usually seen in the uncircumsized male and consists of maceration of the skin from a profuse urethral discharge leading to ulceration of the glans penis and foreskin. Occasionally, cutaneous gonorrhea is seen without an associated urethritis and may be present with irregular purulent ulcerations of the genital skin, probably from infection of an abrasion obtained through intercourse. This condition is to be differentiated from the metastatic skin lesions of gonorrhea mentioned above.

The clinical diagnosis of gonorrhea is substantiated by microscopic examination of a Gram's-stained, thin smear of exudate from the urethra or an ulceration. The finding of gram-negative, kidney bean shaped diplococci within polymorphonuclear leukocytes is sufficient basis for diagnosis (Fig. VII-4). Positive

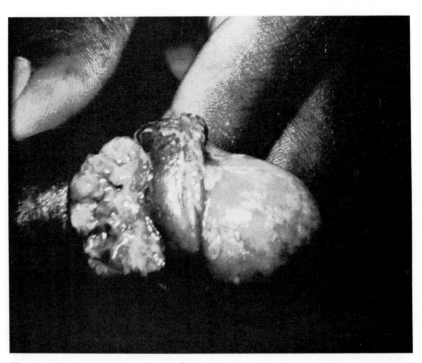

Figure VII-3. Cutaneous Gonorrhea—Gram-negative intracellular diplococci were found in exudate from this lesion. There was no associated urethritis.

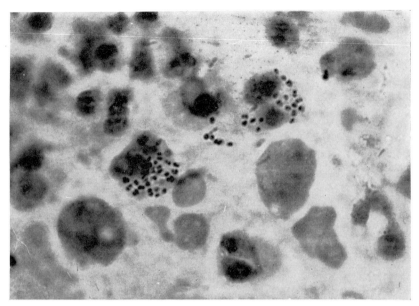

Figure VII-4. Gram-negative intracellular diplococci of *Neisseria gonorrheae*.

smear findings correlate exceedingly well with positive culture results in acute infections in men.

When cultures are used, best results are obtained if a portion of exudate is *directly* inoculated onto chocolate agar or Thayer-Martin medium and incubated under increased CO_2 tension at 35 to 36 degrees centigrade. Specimens for culture are taken with a wire loop from the anterior urethra in males and sterile cotton swab samples from both the anal canal and pharynx in homosexuals. The combination of typical colonies, positive oxidase reaction and demonstration of gram-negative diplococci are sufficient criteria for the presumptive identification of *N. gonorrhoeae*, but fermentation studies are necessary for absolute identification. Fluorescent antibody studies have not been found to be particularly advantageous in the diagnosis of gonorrhea.

Treatment

The decrease in penicillin sensitivity of *N. gonorrhoeae* is well documented internationally, and this has been exceptionally true in Southeast Asia. Despite this fact, penicillin remains the drug of choice since *true* resistance is extremely rare. Gonorrhea is the only bacterial infection of man commonly treated with a large nonrepository dose of antibiotic. The rapid division rate of the gonococcus allows successful therapy with a high blood level of penicillin held for only a short period of time. Although it is still possible to treat most cases of gonorrhea in the U.S. with one single intramuscular dose of 2.4 million units aqueous procaine penicillin, experience indicates that this is inadequate overseas. Two successive daily doses of 2.4 to 4.8 million units of aqueous procaine penicillin G are therefore recommended and 1 gram of oral probenecid may be given simultaneously to delay penicillin excretion and maintain higher blood levels.

In cases of gonorrheal prostatitis or epididymitis, aqueous procaine penicillin G should be given in a dosage of 2.4 million units twice a day for five to seven days. With evidence for septicemia or arthritis, crystalline penicillin G should be given intravenously in a dosage of 10 million units per day for ten to fourteen days.

In persons allergic to penicillin, tetracycline or erythromycin may be used. A loading dose of 1.5 grams should be given followed by 500 mg four times a day for four to seven days.

Of significance in Southeast Asia is urethritis caused by the Mima-Herellae group of organisms. Characteristically, these infections mimic gonorrhea in incubation period, symptoms and morphology on Gram's stain but do not respond to the usual doses of penicillin. Culture studies are necessary for differentiation. Fortunately, complications from *Mima polymorphae* are generally not encountered and infections readily respond to tetracycline. Because of the rarity of true resistance of *N. gonorrhoeae* to penicillin, treatment failure with penicillin can be used as a rough indicator of incidence of infection with the Mima-Herellae group. Positive Gram's stain smears and failure to respond to penicillin may approach 20 percent. Hence, it may be desirable to combine tetracycline with penicillin for treatment of smear positive urethritis under certain circumstances.

Follow-up

Following adequate penicillin therapy, the usual case of gonorrhea is asymptomatic within a 24 to 48 hour period. The patient should be reexamined in approximately one week and any persistent discharge submitted for Gram's stain. If positive, a higher and longer dosage of penicillin or tetracycline may be prescribed. A post-treatment watery or mucoid discharge which is negative on Gram's stain is not uncommon and may be ignored.

Of course, if facilities are available, persistent urethral exudates should be cultured and antibiotic sensitivity determined. Prostatic massage will facilitate obtaining an adequate specimen.

Since it is established that the high doses of penicillin used in the management of gonorrhea will abort incubating syphilis, serologic tests for syphilis should be obtained initially and may be omitted following therapy.

NONSPECIFIC URETHRITIS

Nonspecific urethritis (NSU) or nongonococcal urethritis is not included in the official reporting of venereal disease but constitutes a major portion of military venereal disease clinic effort and case rates may exceed that of gonorrhea. NSU is believed to be sexually transmitted.

Diagnosis

Despite extensive investigation, the cause of most cases of NSU is unknown, although response to tetracycline suggests a microbial etiology. Trichomonas, fungi, mechanical and identifiable chemical irritants cause only a small proportion of NSU and are of minor importance. Although evidence indicates that T-strain Mycoplasma are sexually transmitted, and the Trachoma Inclusion Conjunctivitis and Herpes Virus Hominis agents are potential pathogens, their final roles as causative agents in NSU have not been confirmed. A post-treatment discharge is not uncommon following therapy of gonorrhea with penicillin. This occurs less frequently after treatment with tetracycline.

The time of onset of NSU following sexual exposure is variable, ranging from one to three weeks or longer. The predominate symptom is an itching sensation, independent of urination, in the urethral canal rather than pain as experienced with gonorrheal infection. The discharge is usually thin, not profuse, and clear to milky-white in color. It may be clinically indistinguishable, however, from the urethral discharge of gonorrhea.

Diagnosis is one of exclusion and is determined by microscopic examination of a Gram's stained smear of exudate with failure to find the diplococci of gonorrhea. It is not unusual to find various combinations of gram-negative and gram-positive organisms. Cultures reveal bacteria commonly found on genital skin and are not particularly useful.

Treatment

The majority of cases of NSU tend to clear spontaneously without treatment. It has been impossible to tell with certainty whether recurrences are relapses or reinfections, but recurrences are frequent following treatment. Tetracycline is suggested during the acute phase of NSU and should be given in doses of 500 mg four times daily for five to seven days. Short term treatment should be considered since there is an unproven potential for transmission of untreated NSU.

Follow-up

Periodic Gram's stains should be taken of persistent urethral discharges to ensure gonorrhea has not been overlooked. The prostate gland should be examined. Other antibiotics such as erythromycin may be tried, but long term antibiotic therapy is usually not justified in mild persistent cases of NSU.

SYPHILIS*

The incidence of syphilis has remained relatively stable over the past five years in the military. Also, a number of effective antibiotics are available for cure and late complications are extremely rare. For these and other reasons, efforts towards accurate

---

* Generally, only early syphilis (primary, secondary and early latent) will be discussed in this section.

diagnosis and adequate follow-up have slackened. If relaxation in case finding and reporting continues, however, we may expect a subsequent increase in infectious syphilis and more importantly an increase in congenital syphilis.

Intimate contact is required for transmission of the disease from an infected host to a susceptible individual. Whether the organism can penetrate normal skin or not is a moot point.

Diagnosis

The causative organism, *Treponema pallidum* is a spirochete measuring from six to twelve microns in length. It is extremely susceptible to drying and heat.

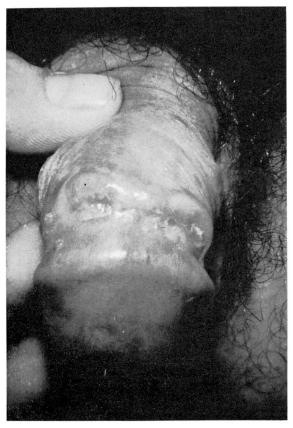

Figure VII-5. Clean, shallow erosions of primary syphilis.

The incubation period of syphilis ranges from ten to ninety days, averaging about three weeks. Classically, a superficial clean, nontender erosion develops at the primary site (Fig. VII-5), soon followed by unilateral, nontender, firm, *rubbery* regional lymphadenopathy. There is a spirochetemia at this time with subsequent development of detectable circulating antibodies.

Primary lesions may occur anywhere on the mucous membranes and cutaneous surfaces but are most common on the penis. They may be multiple. Many times the primary sore is altered by secondary infection leading to a tender, purulent ulceration associated with bilateral tender adenopathy.

The initial sore may heal, but the spirochetemia persists into the secondary stage which may be present with variable manifestations. There is usually generalized lymphadenopathy, possibly with concomitant, mild fever and malaise. There may be alopecia (*moth-eaten* in appearance) usually involving the temporal and occipital regions of the scalp (Fig. VII-6). Whitish patches

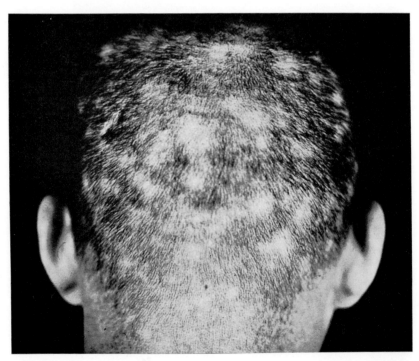

Figure VII-6. *Moth eaten* alopecia of secondary syphilis.

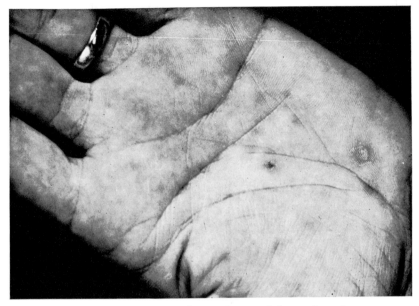

Figure VII-7. Papules of secondary syphilis on the palm.

may be present in the mouth, on the under surface of the foreskin, on the glans penis or in the perianal region. Symmetrical
cutaneous eruptions may appear, ranging from a mild macular
eruption on the trunk to a generalized papular or papulosqua-
mous eruption over the face, trunk and extremities including
the palms and soles (Fig. VII-7). There may be annular indurat-
ed lesions involving the face or moist verrucous lesions involving
intertriginous areas such as the perineum. The spleen may be enlarged.

All lesions of primary and secondary syphilis are considered
infectious and should be dark-field positive. The serologic test
for syphilis becomes reactive soon after the appearance of
lymphadenopathy and should always be reactive in the secondary
stage. If very high titers are present, the prozone phenomenon
may occur giving a falsely non-reactive result. To rule this out,
the serum sample should be diluted 1:100.

It should be pointed out that the primary or secondary stage
of syphilis may be ignored, hidden from the patient or physician (e.g. inside the rectum) or possibly never appear clinically.

A person recently found to have a reactive serology substantiated by a positive FTA-ABS test and no other findings for syphilis should be diagnosed as having early latent syphilis. If a patient is found to have a reactive serology and negative FTA-ABS, the tests should be repeated and the patient evaluated for the significance of a biologic false positive reaction (see Chapter 6).

Generally, spinal fluid examinations are not necessary in the diagnosis of early syphilis. Latent syphilis is differentiated from asymptomatic neurosyphilis by obtaining normal spinal fluid findings; however, an acceptable alternative is longer treatment with an appropriate antibiotic.

Treatment

Penicillin is the drug of choice in the management of syphilis. *T. pallidum* is sensitive to low levels and no resistance has been reported. The organism divides approximately every thirty hours, and for this reason, levels of penicillin must be maintained for relatively long periods (at least ten days) since the drug is effective only during division. This can be achieved by several alternate schedules including 600,000 units of aqueous procaine penicillin G intramuscularly every day for ten days. Benzathine penicillin can be used more conveniently by giving a total of 4.8 million units in two injections one week apart realizing that if an allergic reaction occurs, blood levels will persist for several months.

A convenient *middle of the road* treatment schedule is to give 2.4 million units of procaine penicillin G with 2 percent aluminum monostearate (PAM) IM initially, followed by 1.2 million units every three days for two more doses making a total of 4.8 million units.

The above schedules are recommended for the treatment of early syphilis. In latent syphilis without spinal fluid examination, these schedules should be extended for an additional five to seven days of therapy (e.g. 1.2 million units of PAM for two additional doses three days apart giving a total of 7.2 million units).

Toxic symptoms are very common following the initial injection of penicillin for early syphilis. The reaction, known as the Jarisch-Herxheimer reaction, occurs about six (range: 4 to 14) hours after the start of therapy and may vary from enlargement and tenderness of local lymph nodes to flaring of a generalized cutaneous eruption associated with fever and malaise. The reaction is brief, lasting from a few hours up to eighteen hours. It is not allergy and therefore is not an indication for discontinuing penicillin. Manifestations of the Jarisch-Herxheimer reaction can be minimized or even aborted by treating the patient with erythromycin or tetracycline for forty-eight hours prior to giving penicillin.

In persons who are allergic to penicillin, erythromycin or tetracycline is recommended giving a total dosage of 28 grams over two weeks duration (500 milligrams, four times a day for fourteen days). This treatment period should be doubled in the management of latent syphilis without spinal fluid examination. Since reliance is on the patient to take oral medication, the consequences of inadequate therapy must be emphasized.

Follow-up

A periodic quantitative serologic test for syphilis (STS) is a necessity in follow-up of treated syphilis. Ordinarily, titers will gradually return to normal in persons who are adequately treated. An STS is recommended in one month and then every three months for a period of two years. Relapse or reinfection is detected by an over twofold increase in titer and indicates need for retreatment.

A chronological record of diagnostic methods, diagnosis (including stage), treatment, treatment reactions and periodic serologies is recommended for following treated syphilis. Standard Form 602 (Bureau of the Budget 1952) is used by the military for these record purposes. One copy is placed in the health record of the patient, one is kept by the treating agency and one is given to the patient. In this way, treated syphilis can be accurately followed, and quick reference is available should the problem of a reactive serology come up in the future. Much investigative effort and expense can be saved by using this form.

CHANCROID

The actual incidence of chancroid is difficult to estimate since the diagnosis is often made on clinical inspection alone. It is an uncommon condition in the temperate zones, but becomes very significant in a tropical theater such as Vietnam. The clinical disease is extremely rare in females hindering epidemiological study. Much is yet to be learned regarding the exact nature of chancroid, and simplified methods for establishing the diagnosis are needed.

Diagnosis

The causitive organism, *Haemophilus ducreyi*, is a gram-negative, small, coccobacillary rod. The incubation period of chancroid is short, ranging from three to five days.

Chancroid characteristically presents multiple, painful, purulent ulcerations with undermined borders and associated bilateral, tender lymphadenopathy. The lesions most commonly occur in the uncircumsized under the foreskin and in the sulcus of the penis (Fig. VII-8).

A presumptive diagnosis is made by touching an unaltered lesion with a slide, allowing the exudate obtained to air-dry thoroughly and then submit it to Gram's stain. Pleomorphic organisms are seen in clusters or *school of fish* arrangements (Fig.

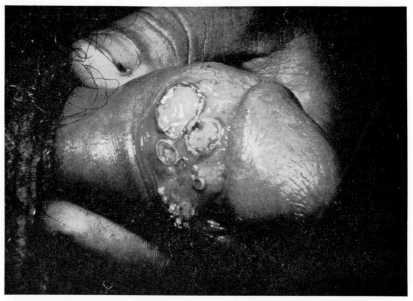

Figure VII-8. Multiple purulent ulcerations of chancroid.

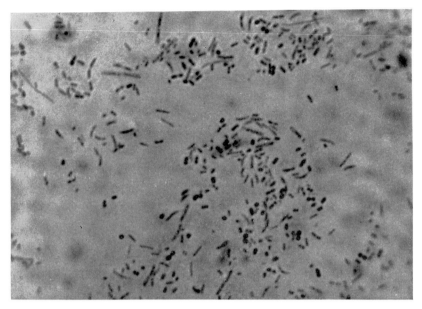

Figure VII-9. *Touch* preparation from an unaltered lesion of chancroid stained with Gram's stain. Note the formation of organisms characteristic of *Haemophilus ducreyi*.

VII-9). These characteristic clusters are broken up if the specimen is not carefully taken and cannot be differentiated from other gram-negative bacteria. Attempts to culture the organism are generally unrewarding.

A small amount of exudate from a lesion may be injected intradermally into the skin of the lower abdomen of the patient. A pustule forms in twenty-four hours, and Gram's stain of carefully-taken exudate will show the typical formation of chancroid organisms. This auto-inoculation procedure may lead to a typical chancroidal ulceration, however.

The most reliable method for proving chancroid is that described by Borchardt and Hoke. Heat-inactivated, patient's serum is inoculated with exudate from a thoroughly cleansed ulceration. After forty-eight hours, parallel arrangement of *H. ducreyi* organisms are seen on Gram stained smears (Fig. VII-10).

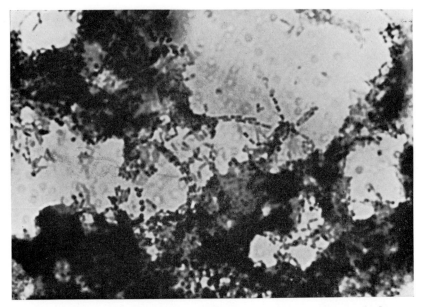

Figure VII-10. Gram stained sample of a patient's serum which was inoculated 48 hours previously with exudate from a cleansed chancroidal ulceration. Note the parallel *(railroad track)* arrangement of Gram-negative streptobacilli characteristic of *Haemophilus ducreyi.*

Treatment

After concurrent syphilis is ruled out by dark-field examination, the treatment for chancroid is oral tetracycline or sulfisoxazole. At least two weeks of therapy is required for cure in most cases, and occasionally this has to be extended to over one month.

Tetracycline is preferred in a dosage of 500 milligrams, four times a day. If incubating syphilis has been missed, this dosage of tetracycline is curative. Allergic reactions are fewer with tetracycline than with sulfonamides. Tetracycline is broader in spectrum, as evidenced by its effective use in urethritis, simple pyoderma and granuloma inguinale.

Sulfisoxazole is adequate in the treatment of chancroid. A loading dose of four grams should be given, followed by one gram, four times a day until complete clearing of the lesions is noted and tenderness in the lymph nodes has subsided. Sulfa drugs do not interfere with incubating syphilis.

Topical therapy is frequently neglected and is very important in the treatment of chancroid. The duration of antibiotic therapy may be decreased as much as one-half with intensive topical treatment.

Frequent compresses with a washcloth or gauze, sloppy wet with plain cool water is recommended for simplicity. These should be applied up to six times a day for about twenty minutes. The lesions should then be adequately dried and a shake lotion containing 3 percent iodochlorohydroxyquinoline applied. Formulation of a suggested shake lotion is as follows:

Iodochlorohydroxyquinoline	3.0
Zinc Oxide	20.0
Talc	20.0
Glycerin	10.0
Water q.s. ad	100.0

This preparation promotes drying. The patient should be instructed to not remove caking from the lesions which will develop after frequent applications.

Follow-up

Antibiotics and topical therapy are continued until complete clearing of all lesions and all signs of inflammation in the affected lymph nodes has disappeared. If sulfa drugs are used, serologic tests for syphilis should be obtained initially and two, four and six months following treatment to ensure that syphilis has not been missed.

LYMPHOPATHIA VENEREUM

This disease, also known as lymphogranuloma venereum, is relatively rare, being more common in the tropics. It is considered a venereal disease; however, little is known about its epidemiology.

Diagnosis

The infectious agent is a large viruslike organism belonging to the psittacosis-trachoma group. There is a variable incubation period of seven to twelve days to appearance of the primary lesion. The primary lesion is a transient vesicle which usually heals in a few days and is frequently unnoticed by the patient. There is then a latent period of two to six weeks before characteristic buboes appear. Hence, enlarged oblong inguinal nodes may be the initial manifestation of lymphopathia and they may be bilateral (Fig. VII-11). If not treated early, these nodes may suppurate and scar.

Lymphopathia venereum is a systemic disease and low grade fever with general malaise accompany the appearance of the lymphadenopathy. A picture of meningitis may appear with stiff neck, headache and lymphocytes in the spinal fluid.

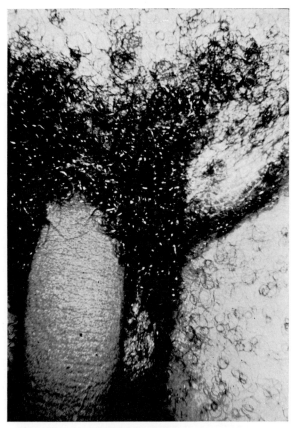

Figure VII-11. Typical lymphadenopathy of lymphopathia venereum.

A Frei test should be performed on patients with suspicious inguinal nodes. Clinical lesions together with a positive skin test are considered adequate for presumptive diagnosis.

Treatment

Tetracycline, 500 milligrams four times a day is recommended in the treatment of lymphopathia venereum. Failures result from inadequate duration of treatment. At least six weeks of therapy is suggested to ensure prevention of late complications such as blockage of lymphatics from the perineal region and rectal strictures.

Sulfisoxazole, one gram, four times a day for a similar period, is also effective.

Follow-up

The patient should be periodically examined to be sure late complications or reactivation of the disease have not occurred. Serologic tests for syphilis should be performed initially and at two, four and six months following initiation of therapy if sulfonamides are used.

GRANULOMA INGUINALE

This disease is extremely rare in the military. Only two cases were diagnosed in the northern section of South Vietnam during 1967 out of over 1,000 venereal disease outpatients seen in the dermatology clinic. Although not proven, venereal transmission is suspected.

Diagnosis

The causitive organism, *Klebsiella granulomatis,* is a gram-negative coccobacillus. The incubation period is possibly one to twelve weeks.

A diagnosis of granuloma inguinale should be entertained if a cutaneous lesion with friable granulation tissue is present in the genital or inguinal regions (Fig. VII-12). No associated adenitis is present unless the lesion is complicated by secondary infection.

Diagnosis is made by crushing a piece of granulation tissue between two slides and staining the material with Wright's stain.

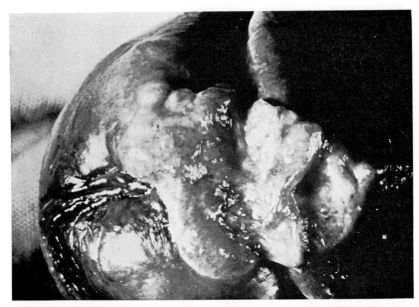

Figure VII-12. Friable, granulomatous lesion of granuloma inguinale in the region of the frenulum on the penis.

Characteristic bipolar staining (closed safety pin) bacteria are seen inside large macrophages.

Treatment

Tetracycline is the drug of choice in the treatment of granuloma inguinale. 500 mg, four times a day should be prescribed for one month or until all evidence of activity has subsided. In addition, topical therapy as outlined for the treatment of chancroid is recommended.

Follow-up

Patients should be periodically examined following treatment to ensure that reactivation of the infection has not occurred.

SIMPLE PYODERMA

Pyoderma or superficial skin infections occur in almost all troops at one time or another, especially in a tropical combat area. Minor scratches, abrasions or lacerations evolve into stubborn, purulent, crusted ulcerations. Factors contributing to bacterial overgrowth and secondary infection include excess heat and humidity and lack of facilities for adequate personal hygiene. Differentiation from venereal disease is required when these lesions occur on the genitalia.

Diagnosis

Studies of the exudate from simple pyoderma reveal nonspecific mixtures of gram-negative and gram-positive organisms. Beta-hemolytic streptococci are commonly found.

Simple pyoderma presents itself as single or multiple purulent

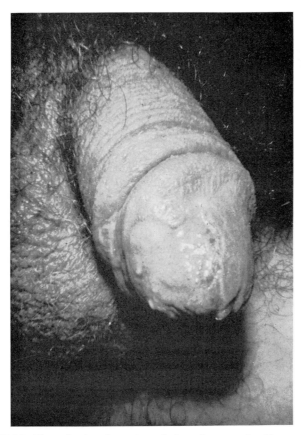

Figure VII-13. Phagedenic ulceration of the glans penis. Gram stains and cultures revealed mixtures of Gram-positive and Gram-negative bacteria.

crusted ulcerations which may or may not be associated with regional adenopathy. Constitutional symptoms are rare.

Laboratory diagnosis is mainly one of exclusion. Gram's stains and dark-field examinations should be done on all suspicious lesions to rule out cutaneous gonorrhea, chancroid and syphilis.

Treatment

Treatment is essentially the same as described for chancroid; that is, oral tetracycline and topical therapy including frequent compresses followed by a topical shake lotion. Simple pyoderma will usually require only a week of therapy for cure as opposed

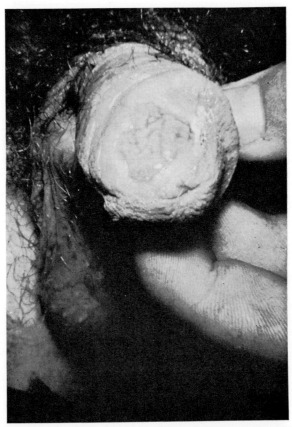

Figure VII-14. Same lesion as seen in Figure 13 after two weeks intensive topical therapy and oral tetracycline.

to chancroid which regularly requires at least two weeks (a therapeutic differentiating point).

Rarely, purulent ulcerations diagnosed as simple pyoderma by the usual criteria, fail to improve or even worsen on the above noted regimen. These are then classified as phagedenic ulcerations (Fig. VII-13) and no antibiotics have been found to be particularly effective. Patients with this condition require hospitalization and intensive topical therapy in the way of very frequent compresses and a drying shake lotion. The lesions heal with moderate scarring (Fig. VII-14).

Follow-up

The patient should be rechecked after one week of therapy and if the lesions are not completely healed, antibiotics may be continued. Serologic tests for syphilis initially and in two and four months following treatment are recommended.

HERPES PROGENITALIS

This not uncommon condition of the genitals causes confusion, unnecessary laboratory efforts and unnecessary concern for the patient in many instances.

Diagnosis

History taking has not been mentioned previously in the management of venereal disease. Much time can be wasted taking unreliable histories with little return. Except for cursory questioning, a detailed history should usually be left up to personnel involved with case finding. Not so with a patient who has herpes simplex. Characteristically, there is a history of recurrent grouped vesicles on an erythematous base localized to one area (Fig. VII-15).

Except for the transient primary lesion of lymphopathia venereum, none of the true venereal diseases present with vesicles. If vesicles are noted, the base of one should be scraped with a curved surgical blade. The material is then placed on a slide and stained with Giemsa's stain for multinucleated epithelial giant cells. The presence of these cells is characteristic for herpes virus infection (Fig. VII-16).

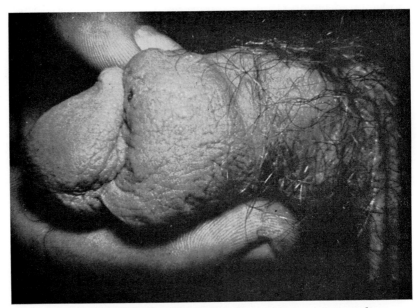

Figure VII-15. Tiny vesicles and swelling of herpes progenitalis.

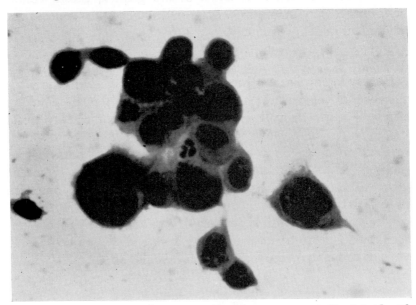

Figure VII-16. Scrapings from a vesicle of herpes progenitalis stained with Geimsa's stain reveal clusters of atypical epithelial cells (positive Tzanck smear).

Occasionally, herpes progenitalis is complicated by secondary infection necessitating Gram stained scrapings and dark-field examinations.

MONILIAL BALANITIS

This condition is frequently seen in the uncircumsized in the tropics. It is also a common complication of broad spectrum antibiotic therapy.

Diagnosis

Diffuse, punctate, brightly erythematous erosions are present over the glans penis (Fig. VII-17). Gram stained scrapings from one of the lesions commonly reveal the large brown, budding spores of a Candida species.

Treatment

Frequent cool compresses followed by a preparation containing nystatin is rapidly effective.

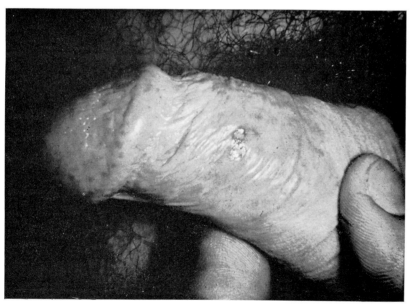

Figure VII-17. An ulceration of chancroid after one week of treatment with tetracycline. Note the numerous lesions of monilial overgrowth on the glans penis.

Follow-up

If monilial balanitis does not rapidly respond to therapy, a search for some underlying disorder such as diabetes should be instituted.

SUMMARY

The occasion arises in the military when one is forced to treat venereal disease without the benefit of clinical and laboratory testing. Should this situation arise, tetracycline in relatively high doses would be the empirical drug of choice.

No *new* or untreatable venereal diseases have been encountered in Southeast Asia unless one would want to place phagedenic ulcerations in that category. As outlined previously, these lesions respond to intensive topical therapy.

REFERENCES

1. Andrews, G. C. and Domonkos, A. N.: *Diseases of the Skin.* Philadelphia, Saunders, 1963.
2. Blair, J. E., *et al.: Manual of Clinical Microbiology.* Bethesda, American Society for Microbiology, 1970.
3. Borchardt, K. A. and Hoke, A. W.: Simplified Laboratory Technique for Diagnosis of Chancroid. *Arch Dermatol,* 102:188, 1970.
4. Brown, W. J., *et al.: Syphilis and Other Venereal Diseases.* Cambridge, Harvard U Pr., 1970.
5. Cooperman, R. S.: VD in Vietnam. *N Engl J Med,* 283:546, 1970.
6. Curtis, J. W. and Carson, T. E.: Dermatoses in Vietnam. *U.S. Navy Medical Newsletter,* 49:16, 1967.
7. Fiumara, N. J. and Lessell, S.: Manifestations of late congenital syphilis. *Arch Dermatol,* 102:78, 1970.
8. Fowler, W.: Studies in nongonococcal urethritis therapy, the long-term value of tetracycline. *Br J Vener Dis,* 46:464-468, 1970.
9. Goltz, R. W.: A dermatologic visit to Vietnam. *Arch Dermatol,* 101:497, 1970.
10. Holmes, K. K., Johnson, D. W. and Floyd, T. M.: Studies of venereal disease: I. Probenecid-procaine penicillin G combination and tetracycline hydrochloride in the treatment of "penicillin-resistant" gonorrhea in men. *JAMA,* 202:461-466, 1967.
11. Holmes, K. K., Johnson, D. W., Floyd, T. M. and Kvale, P. A.: Studies of venereal disease: II. Observations on the incidence, etiology, and treatment of the postgonococcal urethritis syndrome. *JAMA,* 202:467-473, 1967.
12. Holmes, K. K., Johnson, D. W. and Floyd, T. M.: Studies of venereal

disease: III. Double-blind comparison of tetracycline hydrochloride and placebo in treatment of nongonococcal urethritis. *JAMA*, 202: 474-476, 1967.

13. Kerber, R. E., *et al.:* Treatment of chancroid, *Arch Dermatol,* 100:604, 1969.

14. Keys, T. F., Halverson, C. W. and Clarke, E. J.: Single-dose treatment of gonorrhea with selected antibiotic agents. *JAMA,* 210:857-861, 1969.

15. LaChapelle, N. C.: Personal Communication. U.S. Navy Preventive Medicine Unit, Naval Hospital, Oakland, 1971.

16. Lucas, J. B.: Gonococcal resistance to antibiotics, *South Med Bull,* 59, 1971.

17. Medical Services Report: *Nav Med,* 1454.

18. NAVMED P-5052-11A, *Treatment and Management of Venereal Disease.* Dept. of the Navy Publication, Washington, D.C., 1965.

19. Navy Medical Statistical Reporting System: *Statistics of Navy Medicine.*

20. Public Health Service Publication No. 997: *World Forum on Syphilis and Other Treponematoses.* Washington, D.C., U.S. Government Printing Office, 1964.

21. Public Health Service Publication No. 1660: *Syphilis, a Synopsis.* Washington, D.C., U.S. Government Printing Office, 1967.

22. Rook, A., *et al.: Textbook of Dermatology.* Philadelphia, Davis Co., 1969.

23. Sablan, R. G. and Best, W. C.: Febrile response in the Jarisch-Herxheimer reaction. *Arch Dermatol,* 90:293, 1964.

24. Thayer, J. D. and Martin, J. E., Jr.: Improved medium selective for cultivation of N. gonorrhoeae and N. meningitidis. *Public Health Rep,* 81:559, 1966.

25. U.S. Dept. of Health, Education and Welfare, Public Health Service, Health Services and Mental Health Administration, Center for Disease Control, State and Community Services Division, Venereal Disease Branch: *Criteria and Techniques for the Diagnosis of Gonorrhea.* Atlanta, Ga. 30333.

26. U.S. Government Printing Office, Public Health Service Publication No. 859: *Notes on Modern Management of VD.* Reprinted 1962, 22p.

27. White, P. C., Jr. and Blount, J. A.: Venereal disease control in the 2nd Marine division, Camp Lejeune, North Carolina. *Milit Med,* 132: 252, 1967.

28. Youmans, J. B.: *Medical Clinics of North America.* Philadelphia, Saunders, 1964.

CHAPTER 8

ASYMPTOMATIC GONORRHEA

Harry Pariser

THE GONORRHEA RATES in the past ten years have increased four times faster than the population increase, and each year this rate continues to be higher than that of the year before, with no end in sight. I am talking about a big problem. In 1971 about 624,000 cases were reported. Actually the number is probably closer to 2 million new cases. Despite this, there is a surprising complacency about this problem and what is even worse, an attitude of defeatism that nothing can be done about the epidemic of gonorrhea because new infections of gonorrhea are being acquired faster than our ability to treat known cases.

While there are many reasons for this increase in incidence of gonorrhea, probably the single greatest reason for the rapid spread of this infection is the increasing pool of asymptomatic female carriers. Before I discuss this, I would like to stress that there are no signs or symptoms or indeed any combination of signs or symptoms such as vaginal discharge, urinary symptoms, lower abdominal pain and so forth, which are clinically diagnostic of the disease. Conversely, the lack of signs or symptoms does not by any means exclude the diagnosis of gonorrhea. In the Norfolk Venereal Disease Clinic, 80 percent of the females found to have gonorrhea were asymptomatic; that is, they were without symptoms past the usually accepted incubation period of up to eight days after exposure to a known case of gonorrhea. In the female, vaginal discharge is probably more often not due to gonorrhea, whereas in the male, of course, a urethral discharge is most likely to be due to gonorrhea.

How do we go about proving gonorrhea in the female? In the final analysis, whether the woman is symptomatic or asymptomatic, whether the symptoms are related to gonorrhea or not, the diagnosis is usually based upon laboratory findings. Our best laboratory test is the culture. There are over 100 million females in the United States and obviously we can't examine them all. Because of the enormity of the problem, and in order to determine whether a system of priorities is practical the following groups of patients in Norfolk, Virginia were tested consisting of cross sections of different elements of the female population.

A larger series conducted by several clinics and in which the Norfolk Health Department participated showed the following:

TABLE 8-I

ROUTINE EXAMINATION OF FEMALE PATIENTS

	No. Cases	No. Positive	Percent Positive
Contacts of gonorrhea	1,606	527	33.0
Volunteers	833	185	22.2
OB clinics	1,334	49	3.7
GYN clinics	2,285	125	5.4
Family planning clinic	1,903	117	6.1
Routine hospital admissions (USPHS)	1,018	1	.1
Private physician #1—Taylor	500	16	3.2
Private physician #2—Willie	966	10	1.0
Private physician #3—Littlepage	873	18	2.0
Private physician #4—Givens	1,045	10	.9
Private physician #5—Turner	105	1	.9

From the above studies it is apparent that patients named as contacts, those who voluntarily apply to the venereal disease clinics or health centers for examination, female jail patients, patients attending obstetrical and gynecologic clinics and family planning clinics show a sufficiently high percentage of infection to warrant routine examination for gonorrhea.

It will be noted that among private patients the percentage of gonorrhea was low. However, this differed with the type of practice. Gynecologists with patients in the higher socioeconomic brackets uncovered less gonorrhea than gynecologists with patients in the lower socioeconomic classes, although gonorrhea ap-

GONORRHEA SCREENING SUMMARY (FEMALES)
% Positive by Type of Facility Performing Test--FY 1970

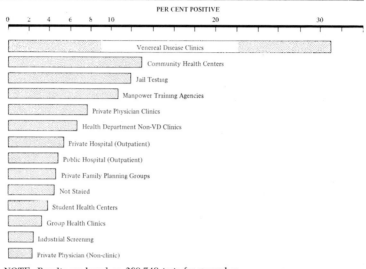

NOTE: Results are based on 269,749 tests for gonorrhea

Figure VIII-1

peared in all groups investigated. Whether or not this small *yield* warrants routine testing by the somewhat cumbersome culture technique in private physicians' offices is a matter of individual decision.

TABLE 8-II

AGE AT TIME OF EXAMINATION AND RESULTS*

	Ob-gyn Clinics		Family Planning		Private Physicians	
	Neg.	Pos.	Neg.	Pos.	Neg.	Pos.
Under 15	22	1	0	0	2	0
15—19	311	29	60	6	133	5
20—24	443	36	137	8	490	12
25—29	256	32	73	3	301	4
30—34	138	4	39	2	139	0
35—39	70	2	18	1	91	0
40—44	50	0	7	0	11	0
45 and over	47	3	3	0	16	0
None given	43	3	0	0	66	1
	1,380	110	337	20	1,249	22

* *From* Pariser, H., and Marino, A. F.: *South Med J* 63:198 (Feb.) 1970, by permission.

It should be noted that over 90 percent of patients with gonorrhea were fifteen to twenty-nine years of age.

I would like to point out that our best diagnostic laboratory procedure, the culture, is positive in about 70 percent of females exposed to known cases of gonorrhea. Of the other 30 percent, undoubtedly some do have gonorrhea, but the culture testing failed to show it. Under any circumstance a female exposed to a patient with gonorrhea should be treated prophylactically whether or not she develops clinical symptoms or has a positive or negative culture. Obviously a better screening procedure would be desirable such as a blood test which could detect active infection. Ideally this test should be sufficiently sensitive to pick up a high percentage of active cases and specific enough not to be positive in a control group such as nuns or priests who presumably should have a negative test. No such blood test is as yet available.

A big disadvantage of the culture screening procedure in the female is the requirement of speculum insertion. This is resisted by many females whose symptoms are not gynecologically related, and therefore many physicians are reluctant to perform this test on a routine basis. Another stumbling block of the culture method for the detection of asymptomatic gonorrhea is that we cannot use an all purpose medium. The gonococcus requires a special medium, the Thayer-Martin medium, which has been devised in such a manner as to encourage the growth of the gonococci and by the addition of antibiotics to eliminate secondary contaminating organisms. A recent modification of the Thayer-Martin medium, the Transgrow medium, has eliminated the need for incubation within a short time, thereby overcoming the big problem of losing the organism during transport.

Recent studies have indicated that the organism is more likely to be recovered from the cervix rather than from other sites. The sites of secondary importance are not the periurethral glands (Skenes) or Bartholin glands as the textbooks state but rather the rectal area.

Over how long a period in her natural course of the disease the untreated female can harbor organisms is unknown. Is it weeks, months or possibly even years?

Another area where the organism may reside asymptomatically is in the pharynx. Within the past few years this site has become to be recognized as an important one. In a recent study by Holmes and his associates they reported that pharyngeal gonorrhea was discovered in 17.2 percent of infected persons exposed by fellatio, and in only 1.4 percent of those denying this activity. In 27 of 47 patients—over one half of those with pharyngeal gonorrhea—the infection was asymptomatic.

Another important reason for the spread of gonorrhea by the asymptomatic female is failure to obtain adequate follow-up after treatment of known cases of gonorrhea. One must remember that treatment is not by any means 100 percent effective. A success rate of between 75 to 95 percent has been recorded with different schedules of antibiotics. One must not assume that because a woman has had an acceptable treatment course or because her symptoms have disappeared she is cured. Also we must realize that there are no sharp clinical signs of cure in the female since most are asymptomatic before treatment.

I would like to point out that there are no absolute criteria of cure. A minimum of two weekly negative cervical and rectal post-treatment cultures and preferably three are desirable to determine probable cure. This post-treatment follow-up procedure has been disputed by some who feel that one seven-day, post treatment, negative culture is adequate proof of cure. Yet we do know that some patients may have a negative test at one week after treatment followed by a positive test the following week or two with no history of reinfection. It is quite true that the longer the post-treatment observational period in an outpatient clinic the more likely the follow-up may be complicated by possible reinfection despite the patient's often unreliable statement that no exposure has taken place. This does present as yet an unsolved dilemma as to what an adequate post-treatment follow up should be in the female. It is indeed paradoxical that many physicians will treat a female exposed to gonorrhea even with a negative culture on the probably correct assumption that she is infected, but will accept one post-treatment negative as the criterion of cure.

The next group of patients I would like to discuss is the asymptomatic male. There are some who dispute the importance or even the existence of a male who has gonorrhea with no urethral symptoms. In our experience we have proved this completely to our own satisfaction. In two studies done in Norfolk, one in 1962 and a second in 1970, it was shown that approximately 12 percent of male contacts of females with gonorrhea showed no discharge, and the infection was discovered only by performing a loop culture. This is done by stripping the urethra, passing a platinum loop into the urethra about one half to three fourths of an inch and gently scraping the surface of the mucosa and immediately planting the specimen on a Thayer-Martin culture medium. It is preferable that the patient not urinate for at least a three hour period before the test is done. In our last study, if we exclude those who fall within the usually accepted incubation period up to eight days, 8.3 percent of these male contacts were asymptomatic from eight to forty-three days after exposure. It becomes somewhat semantic whether we regard this asymptomatic period as a prolonged incubation period or whether we classify these patients as asymptomatic carriers. How long this asymptomatic period can last is unknown since we treated as soon as the infection was discovered.

An additional 3.3 percent of the male contacts had a slight discharge and none of the classical symptoms of pain, burning and frequency on urination. This group did not seek any treatment because they were not sufficiently inconvenienced or disturbed by this minimal discharge. Also, an additional 3.3 percent with frank discharge did not seek treatment primarily because they did not know where to go or were too embarrassed to seek treatment until contacted by one of our epidemiologists, and another 8.3 percent were referred in by their sex partners as the result of interviewing these females. Thus, 26.9 percent of male gonorrhea contacts did not seek treatment and were brought to treatment only following epidemiologic investigation as the result of interviewing female patients for their male contacts. If patients in the asymptomatic or mildly symptomatic groups are promiscuous they constitute a focus of spread greater than their symptomatic counterparts, who, aware of their infection and considerably inconvenienced by it will usually seek medical treatment. Also, these asymptomatic patients, unaware of their infection, are likely candidates for systemic manifestations. It is probable that in the male just as in the female the culture technique does not identify all asymptomatic cases.

I would like to elaborate a little more on the rectal problem both in the male and female because this area is being recognized more and more as a significant source of spread of the infection.

It may come as a surprise to those not engaged in the clinical practice of gonorrhea that the organism can be found in the rectum in a sufficiently large number of cases, to be included in the routine examination for the asymptomatic female carrier. In our experience when this examination was done routinely on the cervix and the rectum of contacts, 40 percent of women with gonorrhea had positive rectal cultures and one fifth of these had a negative cervical culture, i.e. their infection was discovered only as the result of rectal examination. Rectal infection in the female was, in our experience, primarily the result of heterosexual contact in 75 percent of cases. In the male, rectal infection was the result of homosexual practice, as admitted by all but one male with rectal involvement. Often there are no symptoms. I wish to emphasize that after treatment the rectal site as well as the cervical site should show negative cultures before the patient can be declared probably cured.

In the male, as well as in the female, we must not equate the disappearance of signs and symptoms with cure. While it is true that 94 to 95 percent of the males whose signs and symptoms disappear are apparently cured by treatment, about 5 percent of males still show organisms after their symptoms and signs have disappeared. We grant that sometimes it is difficult to determine whether or not this represents a residual infection in which the patient's status has changed from an active infection to a carrier state, or whether this represents an asymptomatic reinfection. Under either circumstance it is important to realize that it is possible for the male as well as the female to harbor organisms asymptomatically after treatment, and he should therefore have post-treatment cultures performed.

In conclusion, I would like to stress four points: one, the most important asymptomatic reservoir of infection is the asymptomatic female; two, the male also can be asymptomatic, a situation at present often ignored or minimized; three, next to the cervix in the female the rectal site is most likely to harbor the gonococcus, and four, patients who practice fellatio should have the pharynx cultured for gonococci.

CHAPTER 9

EXTRAGENITAL GONOCOCCAL INFECTIONS

Charles J. McDonald

"Gonorrhea, commonest of the venereal diseases, is the principal infection caused by the gonococcus *(Neisseria gonorrhoeae)*. From the primary focus in the genital tract, the organism may spread to involve other parts of the body, particularly synovial tissues and serosal surfaces, causing a variety of clinical entities such as arthritis, endocarditis, and meningitis."

William M. M. Kirby (1)

WILLIAM KIRBY's simple, yet concise description of gonorrhea and extragenital manifestations is an appropriate introduction to a discussion which I hope will serve to remind every physician that in this period of rapidly increasing incidence of gonorrhea, he or she must again consider in the differential diagnosis of a multiplicity of disease states the extragenital complications of infection with the organism *Neisseria gonorrhoeae*. This is particularly true when engaged in the examination, diagnosis and treatment of adolescents and young adults.

The rising incidence of gonococcal infections (the number one reportable disease) in the teenage and young adult populations and the ever increasing number of antibiotic resistant strains of *N. gonorrhoeae* are forerunners of a subsequent increase in the incidence of extragenital gonococcal infections. Holmes, and others (2), in reviewing a decade of experience with disseminated gonococcal infections at four cooperating hospitals in Seattle, Washington, found a total of 62 patients having one or more of the systemic manifestations of gonococcal

EXTRAGENITAL GONOCOCCAL INFECTIONS

Primary	*Disseminated*
1. Conjunctivitis	1. Uncomplicated
2. Proctitis	2. Arthritis
3. Oral infections	3. Skin
Stomatitis	4. Perihepatitis
Pharyngitis	5. Peritonitis
	6. Pericarditis and Myocarditis
	7. Endocarditis
	8. Hepatitis

disease. This number, 62, is not very startling or significant in terms of disease incidence when one considers the large numbers of patients with other systemic diseases treated at each hospital during the designated ten-year period. What is startling and significant is the number of patients having these complications who were seen, examined and treated in the last five years of the review. Fifty-seven of the 62 patients were seen during the last half of the decade; 40 of the 57 were actually noted during the last 27 months of the study, and 20 of this 40 were seen in a nine-month period just before and after the conclusion of the review period. These data, in light of the recent rise in the incidence of acute gonococcal infection, clearly demonstrate the coincident rise in the rate of extragenital complications with the rise in incidence of acute gonococcal infection.

Several additional reports (3 to 7) in the medical literature corroborate this data and attest to the fact that the extragenital complications of infection with *N. gonorrhoeae* can no longer be considered rare and insignificant. Bjornberg estimates that 1 to 2 percent of all cases of gonococcal infection seen in his department had manifestations of gonococcal sepsis (8).

EPIDEMIOLOGY

Numerous reports in the literature from medical centers throughout the United States and Western Europe negate Ford's earlier thesis of geography and race, as well as sex, having significant effects on the incidence of extragenital gonococcal infections, particularly arthritis (1, 8 to 10). It is now very evident that the incidence of extragenital gonococcal infections and/or complications parallels the incidence of venereal disease in a given population. Gonorrhea, at present, is epidemic throughout the world and in all segments of society. It is of interest to note that Hart has reported a 2.6 percent rate of asymptomatic infections in a series of private gynecological patients (11).

The increasing incidence of gonococcal infections has been attributed to many unproven factors as a lapse in social and ethical mores, increased promiscuity, male homosexuality and the use of contraceptive pills and the abandonment of other methods of birth control such as the condom, vaginal gels, etc. Any and all of these factors, relevant or irrelevant, are common throughout all segments of all societies; therefore, it is unwise and untrue nowadays to imply that the complications of extragenital disease are confined to a specific racial group (blacks) in a specific geographical area of the world (the Southeastern United States). In fact, is it not fortuitous that the most recent reports detailing experiences with many of the extragenital complications of gonococcal infection have come from the Northwestern United States, Scandanavia and the British Isles (2, 8, 12 to 14).

If one has to single out certain specific social factors and groups of people in whom one is most likely to find disseminated gonococcal disease, it is most probable to find dissemination in (a) adolescents and young adults (ages 14 to 29), (b) females, 75 to 80 percent of all cases, especially during the menstrual period or during pregnancy, (c) in homosexual males and (d) highly mobile populations.

Prior to the use of antimicrobials, the complications of extragenital gonococcal infection were thought to occur more frequently in males. This male predominance has been reversed with most cases now being observed in young females below the age of thirty (15, 16). When seen in males, over 50 percent of those affected are homosexuals. Several reasons for this male-female reversal have been suggested. One concept implies that there has never been a real male predominance, but that gonococcal arthritis is by far the commonest manifestation of disseminated disease, and many males having Reiter's syndrome, with or without genital gonococcal infection, were mistakenly classified as having acute gonococcal arthritis. Proof is thought to lie in the fact that many of the earlier cases of arthritis that developed after acute gonococcal infection did not run the usual course of gonococcal arthritis. A second favored concept is that which relates the female predominance to the very high incidence of asymptomatic gonococcal infection in females. It has been estimated that up to 80 percent of the infected female population are asymptomatic carriers of *N. gonorrhoeae,* whereas less than 20 percent of males with genital infection are asymptomatic. Because most males are symptomatic within three to six days after acquiring a genital infection, they very readily seek medical attention and are treated early in the course of their disease. Females, being relatively asymptomatic, do not often seek early medical attention, i.e. within ten days of the acute infection, and therefore are not treated early. It has been estimated that from ten to thirty days are required after the onset of the primary acute infection to the development of disseminated disease. It has also been estimated that 10 to 15 percent of women who suffer from chronic cervical infection with *N. gonorrhoeae,* develop complications of disseminated disease.

Homosexual males present a similar set of circumstances to that observed in females. Over one half of all male homosexual patients affected with gonococcal proctitis are asymptomatic. Asymptomatic gonococcal proctitis, like cervicitis or vaginitis, goes untreated for long periods of time, over ten to thirty days, thus the asymptomatic infected male homosexual becomes as susceptible to disseminated disease as the asymptomatic infected female.

Primary infection refers to the direct implantation of the organism, *N. gonorrhoeae,* on the affected part. The source of the infection is usually someone other than the victim. Disseminated infection refers to the spread of the gonococcal organism from a primary site in the infected host.

DISSEMINATED GONOCOCCAL INFECTION
General Discussion

Disseminated gonococcal infection probably occurs via two major routes: (a) direct local extension and (b) metastatic spread through the blood stream. Direct local extension in the male occurs by way of the urethra to adjacent organs such as the prostate, and in the female by way of the cervix to the uterus, fallopian tubes and into the peritoneal spaces. This mode of dissemination is very common and results in the greatest number of complications of gonococcal disease. In a small but significant number of persistent gonococcal infections, organisms from the genitalia or other sites of primary infection invade the blood stream and establish metastatic foci in distant organs. In some cases, particularly when serosal surfaces are involved, extragenital manifestations do not appear to arise from the invasion of infective organisms into the symptomatic site, but are probably due to generalized hypersensitivity reactions, or they may arise from the direct toxic effect of viable or nonviable organisms on the tissues (2, 14).

Gonococcal sepsis or disseminated infection via the blood stream present two distinctly different clinical pictures. One offers a rather grave prognosis and involves vital multi-organ systems as the heart, pleura, meninges and skin and is accompanied by high fever. Another clinical state is rather benign and is characterized by a predominance of skin and joint involvement. A multiplicity of organs are affected with the dissemination of gonococcal infection by either of the two routes. The more common sites of involvement are the skin, joints (including the synovial attachments), the perihepatic region, the heart and meninges. As a result, one is able to find in affected persons arthritis, tenosynovitis, skin lesions, pericarditis, myocarditis, valvulitis (endocarditis), perihepatitis and meningitis occurring singly or in various combinations.

Gonococcal Arthritis

Arthritis is the most common of the extragenital complications. It was found in about 1 to 2 percent of cases of gonococcal infection seen in a university medical center (8). There are two basic clinical forms of gonococcal arthritis, but a multiplicity of variations occur (17). In the first type, the *bacteremic form*, arthritis is associated with clinical and bacteriological manifestations of generalized sepsis as fever, chills, skin lesions, polyarticular arthritis and in almost all cases tenosynovitis. On smear and culture of the joint fluid from affected joints, there is no demonstrable evidence of the organism. This finding has led to the descriptive terminology of the so-called *sterile joint.* In the other form, *septic joint form,* generalized septic manifestations are minimal or absent except possibly in a single joint where pain, swelling and an effusion of fluid is often found. *N. gonorrhoeae* can be demonstrated in the joint fluid.

The existence of a bacteriologically *sterile joint,* particularly in the *septic joint form,* is denied by Holmes (18). He believes that organisms can be grown from most joint aspirates if the proper culture conditions as media, temperature, etc. are used. Holmes has suggested that Thayer-Martin medium, although good in most instances for culturing pathogenic Niesseria organisms, is not sufficiently sensitive to isolate all forms of gonococcal organisms that are infecting joint spaces. He has recommended the use of special culture media, such as that described by Bonhoff (19) (overlay medium), as the possible answer to the problem of the identification of gonococcal organisms in *sterile joints.* Awareness of the present status of culture and identification techniques makes it unwise to dogmatically state that the diagnosis of gonococcal arthritis rests on the recovery of organisms from affected joints. Ford considers a diagnosis of gonococcal arthritis invalid unless culture of the aspirate from the joint space is positive for *N. gonorrhoeae.* Most rheumatologists are in accord with the view that negative cultures for *N. gonorrhoeae* do not in themselves rule out gonococcal arthritis in a single or multiple joints. Hypersensitivity or toxicity to the organism and/or its products is sufficient to explain joint symptoms, particularly when polyarticular symptoms occur in the presence of active gonococcal infection.

Gonococcal arthritis has been noted not only as a complication of gonococcal genital infection, but a gonococcal proctitis and pharyngitis (15, 20, 21). The disease progresses very rapidly and is fully developed within two days of the acute onset. In most cases symptoms of primary gonococcal infection are entirely absent. In females arthritis becomes apparent most often during the menses or in pregnancy. If present in pregnancy the patient is probably in the second or third trimester. In the infected male symptoms of arthritis usually arise ten to thirty days after the onset of the acute primary gonococcal infection.

The course of the disease is variable. In 80 percent of patients a migratory polyarthritis is the initial manifestation. Pains most often involve the large joints as the wrists, elbows, knees, ankles and shoulders. The small joints of the hands and feet are rarely involved as are the hip and vertebral joints. If small joint involvement does occur, it is almost never without having one or more of the large joints affected. In 50 percent or greater of patients with joint disease, skin lesions accompany the joint symptoms. Skin lesions, when present, appear during the first four days of the arthritis. In many cases the skin lesions, rather than the arthritis, are the cause of a patient's visit to the physician. In untreated cases after a variable period of time, usually three to five days, the signs and symptoms of joint disease clear completely only to reappear later, localized to a single joint. Localization is accompanied by swelling, pain, tenderness and limitation of motion at the site of involvement. If left untreated, localized joint disease will progress to a frank suppurative arthritis. As is typical of any septic arthritis, narrowing of the joint spaces, erosion of articular surfaces and eventually complete destruction of the involved joint with resultant ankylosis occurs. A few cases resolve spontaneously rather than progressing to frank suppuration and ankylosis.

Tenosynovitis, as manifested by swelling and joint tenderness in the joint region, is very prominent in gonococcal arthritis, appearing in over 50 percent of affected persons. When seen it is usually located at the wrists or ankles. In many instances it is the only evidence of active joint disease. Tenosynovitis occurs more often in active gonococcal arthritis than any other type of arthritis.

The diagnosis of gonococcal arthritis is made in a patient with acute arthritic signs and symptoms not attributable to other conditions and gonococci are demonstrable in the joint fluid or blood, or gonococci are demonstrated in the genitourinary tract or skin lesions with definite improvement noted after antibiotic therapy (17). It will be emphasized again that the isolation of the organism from affected joints is not mandatory for making the diagnosis of gonococcal arthritis. It is generally acknowledged that our limited ability to culture the organism and the absence of adequate quantities of synovial fluid in patients with minimal or no effusions are limiting factors in making a confirmed bacteriological diagnosis of gonococcal joint disease.

THE BACTEREMIC STAGE: In the bacteremic stage polyarthritic symptoms associated with signs and symptoms of sepsis predominate. Chills, fever with temperatures up to 102 to 103°F, tenosynovitis, joint pains and skin lesions all occur within the first three to four days and are indicative of the onset of the bacteremic stage or gonococcemia. The overwhelming experience has been that organisms are rarely isolated from the joints in this stage, but are cultured from the blood and infrequently from the skin. Since the gonococcemia is very transient or intermittent, and if blood cultures are to be obtained as positive proof of infection, they must be taken within three days of the onset of the initial symptoms. If done properly, over 75 percent of blood cultures are expected to be positive in this stage. Infrequently, only patients with associated endocarditis will demonstrate positive blood cultures within the first three to five days of the onset of disease.

SEPTIC JOINT STAGE: The septic joint stage is heralded by the appearance of a solitary, red, hot, swollen, tender and painful joint. There are no associated systemic signs and symptoms. No longer are organisms obtainable from the blood. Purulent material containing *N. gonorrhoeae* is recoverable from 20 to 50 percent of such affected joints. The organism is more frequently isolated from joint fluid containing 30,000 or more cells per mm (3). The average duration of solitary joint symptoms before the proper diagnosis of gonococcal arthritis is made is generally longer in those patients with positive cultures of synovial fluid. Again, the 50 percent or less recovery rate of organisms from joint fluid is probably not related to the absence of active joint infection, but may be related to the absence of normal gonococci and to the presence of abnormal, cell wall deficient or injured gonococci (2). Cultures on a specific hyperosmolar medium are suggested along with the routine and differential media in order to identify the cell wall deficient or injured groups of organisms.

In those persons in whom positive culture evidence of gonococcal infection is not obtainable, prompt resolution of arthritis associated with adequate and appropriate antibiotic therapy is considered compatible with gonococcal infection.

Other laboratory evidences of active disease include an elevation of the synovial fluid white cell count which is nonspecific and is seen in any pyogenic arthritis. Elevation of the synovial fluid count increases as the age of the active joint inflammation increases. Most of the white blood cells in the joint are polymorphonuclear leucocytes. A peripheral blood leucocytosis may or may not occur, blood sedimentation rate is usually normal. There are several serological tests for gonorrhea, such as the gonococcal complement fixation test, etc.; however, these tests are of no use in the diagnosis of gonococcal disease except retrospectively. Using presently available techniques, positive serological examination indicates infection, but does not differentiate between acute and chronic or past infection. The only significant serological test sequence is an initial negative test during the acute stage of the disease and a positive test during or after the convalescent stage. Gonococcal serological titers rise only after the acute stage of arthritis is over. Efforts are presently underway to develop more sensitive and more specific serological tests; field trials of one or more such tests are now in progress.

Radiographic changes, when present, are variable, and most often are nonspecific indicating only the presence of a septic process in the involved joints. Early in the course of the disease the roentgenogram is normal, later on a ground glass appearance of the joint becomes the first manifestation of active disease. This progresses to narrowing and obscuration of the involved joint space and demineralization of small bones. All are indicative of a septic process (9).

Electrocardiographic changes, which will be discussed in detail later, are often present in the bacteremic and acute polyarthritic stage. Gonococcal polyarthritic symptoms and electrocardiographic changes associated with fever in a young male or female often leads to an erroneous diagnosis of acute rheumatic fever.

Before any discussion of gonococcal arthritis is considered complete, its relationship to Reiter's syndrome must be established. A distinct differentiation between Reiter's syndrome and gonococcal arthritis is sometimes very difficult. It is now believed that in the preantimicrobial era, a number of clinical features that were ascribed to gonococcal arthritis are actually features of Reiter's syndrome. This includes the skin lesions of keratoderma blennorrhagica and the arthritis of the *postgonococcal rheumatoid state*. It should be remembered that all patients having Reiter's syndrome do not experience the complete triad of symptoms as urethritis, arthritis and conjunctivitis, and that it is possible for any patient suffering with Reiter's syndrome to have coincidental gonococcal genitourinary tract infection. Several clinical features which differ in the course of each disease should be considered in distinguishing one disease from the other. For example, the arthritis of gonococcal infection is acute and rapidly progressive to a final end point; that of Reiter's syndrome is chronic and recurrent. Gonococcal arthritis has a very prompt response to adequate and appropriate antibiotic therapy. The arthritis of Reiter's syndrome persists in spite of antibiotic therapy. Appropriate antibiotic therapy for gonococcal infection must be emphasized since in many geographical areas, antibiotic resistant strains of gonococci make up 60 percent or more of the organisms causing active infection (22). Also, failure to demonstrate gonococci in joint fluid does not rule out gonococcal arthritis, and therefore should not be used as a major diagnostic determinant.

Treatment of gonococcal arthritis must be immediate and intensive. No distinction should be made in the treatment of patients with positive cultures of the joint fluid and other extragenital sites and those with only arthritis and positive genitourinary tract cultures. Details of a general treatment program for all extragenital infections will be outlined later in this chapter.

Gonococcal Infections of the Heart and Its Coverings

Migratory polyarthritis, fever, leucocytosis, elevated sedimentation rate and an abnormal and unstable electrocardiogram in a young female are considered the *sine qua non* of acute rheumatic fever. It is unfortunate that in most cases of gonococcal infection of the pericardium, myocardium and sometimes the endocardium, the same complex appertains. Since the onset of the antimicrobial era, the number of cases of gonococcal infection of the heart and its covering has been reduced. However, again with the increasing incidence of acute gonococcal infection there is an expected rise in the incidence of myocardial, pericardial and the most dreaded of gonococcal infections, endocardial disease.

Gonococcal Endocarditis

Gonococcal endocarditis, unrecognized and untreated early in its course, offers a very grave prognosis. Prior to the antibiotic era, gonococcal endocarditis accounted for up to 26 percent of the reported cases of bacterial endocarditis.

Davis (23) credits Thayer and Blumen (24) for first reporting in 1896 the recovery of the gonococcus from the blood of a patient having endocarditis. Since then over 200 cases have been reported in the literature, most being reported prior to 1942 or prior to the beginning of the penicillin era. The most recently reported cases are those of Holmes (2).

The presenting signs and symptoms are usually noted in the joints with most patients complaining of a very severe polyarthritis. Several days to weeks after the beginning of joint pains, the patient begins to complain of chills, malaise, chest pain and dyspnea on exertion. Physical examination at this stage of disease reveals a high fever 101 to 103°F, a rapid pulse rate, an abnormal blood pressure and pathological murmurs. The abnormal blood pressure and the pathological murmurs assume the characteristics which are associated with the specific valvular abnormality, i.e. involvement of the aortic valve leading to aortic regurgitation is characterized by a low diastolic pressure, wide pulse pressure and a loud diastolic parasternal murmur. In most patients these signs and symptoms lead to the improper clinical diagnosis of acute rheumatic fever; thus the patient is treated with nonspecific measures consisting of bed rest and high doses of salicylates. In such unfortunate cases the rapidity of progression of the disease and the failure to initiate immediate antibiotic therapy leads to severe sequela, such as irrepairably damaged heart valves, and death. Death in untreated cases occurs within ten days to two weeks after the onset of the endocardial disease.

Skin lesions probably related to septic emboli from valvular vegetations may appear during the acute stage. They do not differ in appearance from similar lesions seen in other forms of septic valvulitis.

Laboratory findings are nonspecific. The white blood cell count is normal, the sedimentation rate is normal or only slightly elevated. The electrocardiogram may be normal or show changing nonspecific patterns. Blood cultures are sometimes sterile during the polyarthritic stage becoming positive with the onset of endocardial involvement. As is the case in other forms of endocardial disease, multiple blood cultures are often required to obtain a single positive culture. Because of the serious sequela of gonococcal endocarditis and the difficulty encountered in isolating the causative organism in suspected patients, it is probably wise to initiate specific antibiotic therapy immediately after an adequate number of blood cultures has been obtained.

Examination of necropsy material has demonstrated that the left side of the heart is most frequently involved with disease, and the aortic valve is the most frequently involved valve. Other valves, i.e. mitral, pulmonic and tricuspid can be involved alone or in various combinations. Vegetations, thickening, shortening and perforations of valve leaflets can be found. A myocarditis may accompany the endocarditis.

Gonococcal Myocarditis and Pericarditis

Although disease of the myocardium and pericardium is observed more often in disseminated gonococcal infection than endocardial disease, the consequent involvement of the myocardium and pericardium leads to less serious disease sequela. In most patients pericardial and myocardial infection are noted as a result of electrocardiographic examination; rarely are patients symptomatic, and rarely do they demonstrate positive cardiac physical findings. Arthritis is usually the presenting symptom which brings the patient to the physician. Electrocardiographic examination in two of five of Vietzkie's patients, all of whom presented gonococcal arthritis, and eight of seventeen of Holmes' patients with disseminated disease, seven of whom had arthritis, showed abnormal electrocardiographic findings (2, 25). Similar findings have been noted in other reported series. The electrocardiographic changes are characteristic of those observed in any type of acute pericarditis, particularly purulent, and include a prolongation of the PR interval, inverted T waves and elevation and coving of ST segments in any or all leads (26 to 28). These electrocardiographic changes revert to normal with adequate antibiotic therapy. The electrocardiographic findings which are observed are thought to arise from active myocardial disease, *toxic myocarditis,* that is probably secondary to pericardial inflammation. *Toxic myocarditis* implies that disease of the myocardium does not necessarily arise from direct involvement of muscle tissue by *N. gonorrhoeae,* but arises from toxins or by-products of the infective organism in surrounding tissues.

Again, to reemphasize a point made earlier but which cannot be overemphasized, the migratory polyarthritis, fever, chills and electrocardiographic abnormalities of acute gonococcal arthritis and pericarditis-myocarditis resemble those of and are often confused with rheumatic fever. Rheumatic fever in such cases is ruled out by the lack of disease response to bed rest and salicylates and on occasion the development of septic joint disease. Failure to make an early diagnosis of pericardial-myocardial disease does not lead to sequelae of the magnitude of endocardial disease.

Gonococcal Abdominal Infections

The infection of abdominal organs with *N. gonorrhoeae* can occur as a result of gonococcal bacteremia or as a result, especially in the female, of direct spread of the organism from the genital organs to contiguous structures.

Gonococcal Perihepatitis

In 1930 Curtis first described his clinical experiences with several cases of *violin-string* or banded adhesions between the liver and the anterior abdominal wall in women suspected of having gonococcal pelvic disease (29). He became aware of this phenomenon during a customary practice of his, the routine intra-abdominal examination of all the palpable organs in females undergoing pelvic surgery. He was so impressed with the frequency of his findings of banded right upper quadrant adhesions in patients with evidence of gonococcal disease, i.e. salpingitis, that he began to *anticipate* tubal disease whenever his palpating hand found characteristic adhesion bands on exploration of the anterior surface of the liver. Because he frequently found similar adhesive disease in patients with chronic upper abdominal pain, he concluded that many "female patients with symptoms suggestive of gallbladder disease or pleurisy may be suffering from liver-abdominal wall adhesions complicating a pelvic gonorrheal infection."

In 1934 Thomas Fitz-Hugh described three cases of acute gonococcal peritonitis in women and felt that these three women demonstrated the acute and early manifestations of the disease described in the end stage by Curtis (30). In 1936 Fitz-Hugh coined the term *acute gonococcic perihepatitis* for the syndrome of right upper quadrant abdominal pain in young women (31). Subsequently, the syndrome became known as the Fitz-Hugh Curtis syndrome.

Until the report of Kimball in 1970, acute gonococcal perihepatitis was thought to exist only in females (32). A plausible explanation for this female predominance is thought to arise in the ease of passage of infecting organisms from the female lower genital tract through the fallopian tubes and paracolic gutter to the subphrenic space. In males there is no comparable anatomical continuity between the genital organs and the abdominal cavity, therefore, the existence of this type complication would be rare in males. In males it is postulated that perihepatitis occurs as a result of bacteremia or spread from the genitals via the retroperitoneal lymphatics.

The clinical signs and symptoms of perihepatis may simulate acute cholecystitis, nephrolithiasis, perinephric abscess, pyelonephritis, hepatitis, pneumonia, pleurisy, perforated peptic ulcer and subphrenic abscess (30). Affected patients complain of severe anterior right upper quadrant pain; the pain is usually sharp in nature, and it may be referred to the right shoulder. Occasionally, pain may be referred to both shoulders. Nausea and belching are common. Vomiting is less frequent, but does occur in some patients. In most patients it is possible to obtain a previous history of lower abdominal pain, with or without fever, leukorrhea and dysuria, all suggestive of pelvic inflammatory disease. There is normally a three to four week period of quiescence of the pelvic inflammatory disease before the acute onset of severe upper abdominal pain. Coughing, sneezing, straining, laughing and twisting movements of the trunk often aggravate the pain (31).

The physical findings in the acute stage include a slightly elevated temperature; on infrequent occasions it rises to 102°F. A moderate amount of abdominal distention may be noted. A to and fro *new snow* friction rub sometimes is heard over the anterior abdominal wall; peristaltic sounds are normal to diminished. Marked tenderness and rigidity are noted in the anterior and lateral right upper quadrant. A positive Murphy's sign may be present. The liver may be enlarged. Only minimal tenderness and rigidity are noted in the lower abdominal quadrants (31, 32).

A pelvic examination at this time may or may not be compatible with active pelvic inflammatory disease. However, urethral and cervical cultures are usually positive for gonococcus.

In untreated cases all symptoms subside in three to six weeks, then the chronic stage as defined by Curtis begins.

During the acute phase a leucocytosis is not evident, although there may be a shift to the left in the differential white cell count. The sedimentation rate is high even in the absence of signs and symptoms of acute disease.

X-rays during the acute phase will sometimes demonstrate nonvisualization of the gallbladder. Subsequent studies will show normal gallbladder function.

Liver biopsy during the acute phase shows normal liver architecture.

A direct visual examination of the affected area shows inflammation of the peritoneum of the overlying liver surface and of the adjacent abdominal wall. Blood vessels at the site are injected, and a granular or flaky grayish exudate is seen to overlie the liver capsule. *N. gonorrhoeae* can in some cases be cultured from the surface exudate. Histologically, gonococcal perihepatitis differs from gonococcal hepatitis in that the inflammation is usually confined to the liver capsule, and in most cases open liver biopsy shows normal liver architecture. Infrequently, the liver adjacent to the affected area shows mild inflammatory changes in the liver parenchyma. This minimal involvement is to be distinguished from active parenchymatous involvement of the liver with blood-bone spread of gonococcal infection. The inflammatory liver disease associated with acute perihepatitis, if observed, is always confined to the outer parenchymatous zone and is traceable as an extension from the affected overlying liver capsule. Other differentiating features are the normal liver function studies obtained in patients with acute perihepatitis.

Untreated cases apparently lead to no significant sequela other than the *violin-string* adhesions of Curtis. The significance of the disease lies in its recognition and the need to differentiate it from more serious acute abdominal disease. As an aid to differentiating perihepatitis from other upper abdominal disease, Kimball stresses several features that are characteristic of the typical patient having perihepatitis. "She is a young female with signs and symptoms of acute cholecystitis and a recent purulent genitourinary tract infection" (32).

Gonococcal Hepatitis

Gonococcal hepatitis is thought to arise as a result of gonococcal bacteremia. It may occur as an isolated entity or may be accompanied by fever, a dermatitis and arthritis. Tests of liver function are abnormal in a large number of persons known to have disseminated gonococcal disease. At least 50 percent of the patients having positive blood cultures or skin lesions when examined by Holmes had abnormal liver function tests (2). Others have reported jaundice accompanying other evidence of disseminated gonococcal infection (33, 34). Gonococcal hepatitis much like perihepatitis appears not to lead to serious sequela. As is true of gonococcal perihepatitis, gonococcal hepatitis' significance also lies in the need to distinguish this disease from other more serious forms of hepatitis.

Gonococcal Peritonitis

Gonococcal peritonitis is somewhat rare as a specific entity, and this is quite surprising in view of the rather high incidence of pelvic inflammatory disease that is observed in females after acute gonococcal genitourinary tract infection. The disease is characterized in its early stage by mild abdominal discomfort followed almost immediately by fever, nausea with or without vomiting, abdominal pain accentuated in the lower abdominal quadrants and a rather profuse vaginal discharge.

The physical examination is typical of that observed in any patient with abdominal peritonitis of bacterial or chemical causation. Treatment with the appropriate antibiotic leads to prompt clearing of disease in five to seven days.

The disease is rare in preadolescent females.

The rarity of the disease in preadolescent females in the face of an ideal vaginal pH of 7 and a thin, delicate vaginal wall is probably related to the absence of endocervical glandular structures, the harbingers of *N. gonorrhoeae* in postadolescent females (35).

Gonococcal Meningitis

Meningitis is a rare complication of disseminated gonococcal infection (36 to 39). Holmes has found only 14 documented cases in the literature (2). When it occurs, it is difficult to distinguish from acute meningococcal meningitis. Sugar fermentation reactions after culture of the organisms is the only satisfactory method of distinguishing meningeal disease caused by *N. gonorrhoeae* from that caused by *N. meningitidis*. Spread of

N. gonorrhoeae to the meninges probably occurs via the blood stream, therefore, one can expect to observe skin lesions and polyarthralgias in an affected individual. About 50 to 60 percent of the reported cases of gonococcal meningitis demonstrate either or both, i.e. arthralgias and skin lesions. This is in distinct contrast to the 2 to 10 percent occurrence of arthralgias in cases of meningococcal meningitis. Other signs and symptoms of gonococcal infection of the meninges are those characteristic of meningitis from any cause and include fever, chills, headache, photophobia, nausea, vomiting, agitation and tremor. Examination of the spinal fluid demonstrates a leucocytosis, 3000 to 5000 WBC/mm^3, most of which (75 to 85 percent) are neutrophils, an elevated protein and a low sugar content. Positive cultures of *N. gonorrhoeae* can be obtained from the spinal fluid in the acute stages. Blood cultures may or may not be positive.

Prompt recovery from the infection occurs with adequate, specific antibiotic therapy, however, it is interesting to note that prior to the introduction of antimicrobial therapy over 60 percent of patients affected with gonococcal meningitis recovered without residual disease. This again is in distinct contrast with the experience noted in cases of active *N. meningitis* infection of the meninges.

Cutaneous Gonococcal Lesions

Gonococcal skin lesions are the second most common manifestation of disseminated disease, and are almost always associated with those complications of gonococcal disease that result from blood borne dissemination of *N. gonorrhoeae*. Skin lesions are associated with the bacteremic form of gonococcal arthritis, meningitis, endocarditis and hepatitis. Infrequently, skin lesions occur without other manifestations of other types of disseminated gonococcal infection. Skin lesions associated with positive blood cultures have been described in a male patient having no other signs of dissemination after prostatic massage (14).

Vidal has been credited with the first description of skin lesions in gonorrhea (40). These lesions were observed in a patient with gonococcal arthritis. Over one third of patients having acute gonococcal arthritis will demonstrate some type of skin lesion.

There are three basic types of skin lesions seen in disseminated gonococcal disease: (a) vesicopustular lesions on an erythematous base, (b) hemorrhagic papules and (c) bullae (41 to 44). They may simulate and must be differentiated from lesions caused by meningococci, the skin lesions of drug reactions, rheumatic fever, subacute bacterial endocarditis, rheumatoid arthritis, systemic lupus erythematosus, cutaneous allergic vasculitis, periarteritis nodosa and typhoid fever.

The skin lesions of disseminated gonococcal infection tend to occur within the first three to five days of the blood bone spread of disease. Often they appear as the first definitive sign of disease and very often are the cause of the patient's visit to a physician. Skin lesions tend to appear in crops with a few new lesions developing each day during the acute stages of disease. Some lesions may be solitary, or they may be few in number. They usually localize over the joints of the extremities, and may on occasion be symptomatic with tenderness being elicited over the actual lesion.

Most lesions evolve through the development of a tiny red papule to a pustular or vesicopustular stage, all surrounded by a macular red base, and then undergo spontaneous involution in four to five days. Most will leave small scars after developing purpuric or necrotic central regions just before clearing. Blood cultures in 50 percent or more of patients with skin lesions will be positive for *N. gonorrhoeae,* an almost certain indication of bacteremic spread of the disease. Smears and cultures of active skin lesions may or may not yield positive gonococcal cultures. The culture or organisms from skin lesions definitely occurs less often than from blood cultures in disseminated disease. Kahn has demonstrated gonococci and gonococcal antigens in gonococcal skin lesions using an immunofluorescent technique (45). The inherent difficulty in performing this procedure makes it impractical for general use.

The histopathological examination of a typical skin lesion has been described by Ackerman (42). There was an arteritis with a dense aggregate of mononuclear and polymorphonuclear white cells surrounding an arteriole. There were polys containing gram-negative diplococci lying within the arteriolar lumen. A few diplococci were seen in the wall of several blood vessels. A pustule was located in the epidermis just above the inflamed arteriole.

PRIMARY EXTRAGENITAL GONOCOCCAL INFECTIONS

Primary extragenital infections are thought to arise as a result of the direct implantation of the organism, *N. gonorrhoeae,* on the affected part. The source of the infection is another externally affected part of another person and is usually associated with intimate person to person contact. Occasionally an individual may infect himself such as genitals to eye via digits, etc. The vascular system and contiguous structures are not involved in the spread of primary infection.

Gonococcal Oral Infections

Numerous reports of primary gonococcal infection of the oral cavity have been published, however, this specific form of oral infection apparently continues to be overlooked as a cause of stomatitis, parotitis, pharyngitis and tonsillitis (20, 46 to 49). Gonococcal infection of the oral cavity should take on a more significant role in the transmission of primary infections with the changing patterns of sexual behavior and the increasing incidence of homosexuality. Metzger has described a case of gonococcal arthritis secondary to gonococcal pharyngitis (21).

Most cases of primary oral gonococcal infection have been observed soon after some form of orogenital exposure (fellatio and cunnilingus), although Schmidt does call attention to the presence in the medical literature prior to the onset of the twentieth century (46) of a description of gonococcal stomatitis in the newborn.

Most early reports in the literature circumstantially incriminated the gonococcus as a cause of primary oral infection, i.e. history of orogenital contact in a patient having oral complaints and positive findings of gonococcal infection in the sexual partner. Fiumara and others in 1967 reported one definite case of gonococcal pharyngitis (bacteriologically confirmed) and two other probable infections in a group of homosexual males (20). This report was followed in 1970 by Metzger's report of primary gonococcal pharyngitis complicated by arthritis in a male who admitted to orogenital contact with a woman and man fourteen and six days respectively before the start of his illness (21). There was no history of coitus with the female. Positive cultures of *N. gonorrhoeae* were obtained in this case from the throat, blood and temporomandibular joint.

The symptoms attributable to primary gonococcal oral infection are variable and in most individuals are dependent on the anatomical location of the infection. Itching, burning, soreness and dryness of the mouth, accompanied by headache, fever and chills may be the presenting complaint in gonococcal stomatitis. The patient often experiences difficulty in opening and closing the mouth and in eating solid foods. In cases of tonsillitis and/or pharyngitis, a persistent dry mouth and sore throat, accompanied by headache, fever and chills may herald the onset of the disease. In cases associated with a migratory polyarthritis, the disease may simulate acute rheumatic fever, serum sickness, subacute bacterial endocarditis, Reiter's syndrome and collagen vascular diseases.

An examination of the oral cavity is variable and in cases of stomatitis often reveals a tender, fiery red or whitish-yellow, oral mucous membrane and areas of greenish-yellow patches, yellow exudates, linear or flattened eroded lesions, chafed lips, and yellowish to grey pseudomembranes that tend to be quite friable when scraped off. Aphthous like lesions may be noted on the mucous membranes. The salivary secretions are thick and ropy and reduced in amount. The patient may or may not have associated genital complaints.

In pharyngeal and/or tonsillar disease, the pharynx shows patchy to diffuse erythema and edema. The anterior and posterior tonsillar pillars and uvula are swollen and red. There may be small clear vesicles or discrete pustules over the uvula and anterior tonsillar pillars. One or both tonsils may be enlarged and inflamed with a mucopurulent yellow to white discharge located in the crypts. The anterior cervical nodes may be enlarged.

Cultural techniques to isolate the gonococcal organism must rely heavily on the use of various specific bacteriological differentiations of the offending organism from the oral cavity. A large number of nonpathogenic as well as pathogenic Neisseria such as gonococci, meningococci, catarrhalis, sicca, flava and perflave may inhabit the oral cavity. Morphologic identification as to size, shape and location of the organisms is unreliable. Specific selective growth media such as the Thayer-Martin is helpful in this regard, eliminating from consideration all nonpathogenic Neisseria. Sugar fermentation techniques aid in differentiating gonococci and meningococci.

Gonococcal infection of the oral cavity must be differentiated from erythema multiforme with or without associated herpes simplex infection, aphthous stomatitis, tonsillitis and erosive or bullous lichen planus. A very rapid response of disease to specific antibiotic therapy (in one to three days) is characteristic of gonococcal infection of the oral cavity and tends to eliminate from consideration those diseases mentioned above.

Gonococcal Eye Infection

Along with the increasing incidence of gonococcal genital infection there has been an increasing number of reports of cases of primary gonococcal infection of the eye. Some have been reported in newborns (ophthalmia neonatorium), others have been reported in teenagers and young adults.

Primary gonococcal infection of the eyes of newborn infants, ophthalmia neonatorium, obtained during the infant's passage via the birth canal of an infected mother, has been almost nonexistent since the introduction of the Crede technique which consists of installing a dilute solution of silver nitrate into the conjunctival sac of each infant at birth. More recently the practice of installing antibiotics such as penicillin into the conjunctival sac of infants to prevent gonococcal eye infection at birth, has gained favor.

The effectiveness of installing silver nitrate solution in the eyes of infants at birth for the prevention of gonococcal disease has recently been challenged (50). Abandonment of this technique of prevention for a method of direct installation of specific antibiotics into the conjunctival sac has been suggested. However, the increasing incidence of antibiotic resistant organisms makes this practice also questionable.

In two cases of gonococcal eye infection reported by Thatcher the routine installation of silver nitrate drops into the eyes of each infant at birth did not prove sufficiently effective to prevent ophthalmia neonatorium from occurring, thus indicating the ineffectiveness of, or at best, the partial effectiveness of this form of prophylaxis in some gonococcal infections.

Gonococcal conjunctivitis in other than neonates is the result of direct inoculation of the gonococcus onto the conjunctivae either by direct transfer by fingers, self-infection or infection from an infected intimate acquaintance. Primary gonococcal conjunctivitis, like primary gonococcal infection of the genitals, has an incubation period of from one to six days after which the infection becomes rapidly progressive and if left untreated eventually involves contiguous eye structures. The end result of untreated disease is corneal ulceration. Corneal ulceration occurs with such rapidity that immediate diagnosis and treatment is imperative in gonococcal conjunctivitis.

The disease may manifest early as an indolent conjunctival infection, as seen in one recent case on the pediatric service (a six month old female infant), demonstrating minimal erythema, edema and a serosanguinous then yellow-white exudate in the conjunctivae, or as in most cases, may be present initially with a severely inflamed, red, swollen and infected conjunctivae exuding a purulent creamy white to yellow-white discharge. Most often the initial signs of gonococcal disease are confined to one eye. One to six days later the other eye becomes involved. If left untreated, or if treated with an inappropriate antibiotic, corneal ulceration, hypophyon and early neovascularization of the cornea with its attendant loss of visual acuity may occur within a five to six day period (50 to 52).

TREATMENT OF EXTRAGENITAL GONOCOCCAL INFECTION

Prior to the recent upsurge in venereal disease infections, a single dosage of short-acting penicillin as low as 300,000 units was expected to cure any case of gonorrhea. However, it is becoming increasingly evident throughout the world that the emergence of drug resistant strains of gonococci has called for higher and higher dosages of drug to effect a cure. Presently the U.S. Public Health Service recommends a single intramuscular dosage of 4.8 million units of a short-acting penicillin for the treatment of uncomplicated gonococcal infection in a male as well as in a female with uncomplicated disease. If the present trend continues this dosage regimen is destined to rise higher and higher. Some authorities add 1 to 2 gm of probenecid to the recommended penicillin dosage regimen to delay its excretion and maintain a high blood level of penicillin for a longer period of time (53). It must be emphasized that high blood levels of penicillin for short periods of time are desirable for the treatment of gonococcal infection, therefore, the long acting penicillins which are designed to provide low blood levels of drug over a prolonged period of time are contraindicated in the treatment of gonococcal infection.

Gonococcal proctitis appears to be much more difficult to treat than gonococcal infection of the genital tract. Since approximately 49 percent of females having genital gonorrhea who have been examined rectally show positive rectal cultures (4), and the percentage is probably even higher in the male homosexual population, it is wise to treat both these groups with higher dosages of drugs than are presently recommended by the U.S. Public Health Service.

For the treatment of the complications of disseminated gonococcal infection or other than primary genital disease, no set regimen has been advocated. A single author reporting on his experience in five different patients having the same complication of disseminated disease will probably report five different therapeutic regimens.

Presently, in the treatment of disseminated gonococcal infection as little as 1.2 million units of procaine penicillin G given daily for five to seven days has effected a cure. However, current practices dictate that from 3 to 10 million units of aqueous or procaine penicillin G be given parenterally for ten or more days to effect a cure. In most complications clinical improvement will be seen within twenty-four to forty-eight hours of instituting specific antibiotic therapy. For several unrelated reasons many physicians have abandoned the syringe (penicillin) in favor of oral antibiotic therapy. Many penicillin-resistant strains have been found to be responsive to single or multiple dosages of broad spectrum antibiotics (54 to 56). Of the oral penicillins, ampicillin appears to be the drug of choice, particularly when combined with at least 1 gm of probenecid daily (57).

The tetracyclines have proven somewhat effective in treating anogenital gonococcal infection and penicillin-resistant infections. Doxycycline in a single dosage of 200 to 300 mgs is thought to be effective in controlling noncomplicated, gonococcal infection, however, here again in treating the complications of disseminated infection treatment should probably be continued for ten or more days for more effective cure. The other tetracyclines should be used in a dosage of 2 gms or more daily for at least ten days. Spectinomycin hydrochloride, a new injectable antibiotic, has been shown to be effective in curing up to 100 percent of male and female patients when used in single dosages of 2 to 4 gms (58).

For patients allergic to penicillin, oral tetracyclines in dosages of 2 to 3 gms daily for ten or more days is considered adequate treatment.

The signs and symptoms of most complications or of primary gonococcal disease when treated adequately will begin to subside within 24 to 48 hours and are absent in seven to eight days. Rarely, in some cases of gonococcal arthritis and endocarditis, signs of acute disease will persist for one month or more. Any damage to the joints and heart valves that has occurred prior to the initiation of antibiotic therapy is permanent and cannot be reversed. Replacement of affected valves may offer the only relief of severe cardiac damage in cases of endocardial disease.

Joint aspirations may be required to aid in clearing affected joints. The role of active or passive motion of affected joints in the acute stage of disease has yet to be adequately assessed.

Infection of the conjunctivae presents a special problem. Systemic therapy should be supplemented by topical therapy such as tetracycline in oil or chloramphenicol given at very frequent intervals, i.e. every fifteen to thirty minutes throughout the day for five to seven days. Saline irrigations should supplement the antibiotics at about equal frequency.

The role of early diagnosis and adequate, appropriate treatment of the complications of disseminated gonococcal infection and primary extragenital infections in the prevention of serious sequela cannot be overemphasized. It is to be remembered that gonococcal infections diagnosed early and treated early are curable diseases.

REFERENCES

1. Kirby, W. M. M.: Diseases caused by Neisseria—gonococcal disease. In Beeson-McDermott and Cecil-Loeb: *Textbook of Medicine,* 11th Ed. Philadelphia, Saunders, 1963, p. 196-200.
2. Holmes, K. K., Counts, G. W. and Beaty, H. N.: Disseminated gonococcal infection. *Ann Intern Med,* 74:979-993, 1971.
3. Molin, L.: Gonorrhea in 1968. *Acta Derm Venereol,* 50:157, 1968.
4. Schroeter, A. L. and Pazin, G.: Gonorrhea. *Ann Intern Med,* 72:553-559, 1970.
5. Complications of gonorrhea. *Br Med J,* 3:420, 1970.
6. New problems and old ones back again. *Lancet,* 2:872-873, 1970.
7. Hansen, T., Burns, R. P. and Allen, A.: Gonorrheal conjunctivitis: an old disease returned. *JAMA,* 195:1156, 1966.
8. Bjornberg, A.: Benign gonococcal sepsis. A report of 36 cases. *Acta Derm Venereol* (Stockh), 50:313-316, 1970.
9. Ford, D. K.: Gonococcal arthritis in arthritis and allied conditions. In Hollander, J. L. (Ed.): 6th Ed. Philadelphia, Lea and Febiger, 1960, p. 995-1000.
10. Ford, D. K. and Rasmussen, G.: Relationships between genitourinary infection and complicating arthritis. *Arthritis Rheum,* 7:220-227, 1964.
11. Hart, M.: Gonorrhea in women. *JAMA,* 216:1609-1611, 1971.
12. Haim, S. and Merzbach, D.: Gonococcal penile ulcer. *Br J Vener Dis,* 46:336-337, 1970.
13. Cowan, L.: Gonococcal ulceration of the tongue in the gonococcal dermatitis syndrome. *Br J Vener Dis,* 45:228-231, 1969.
14. Wolff, C. B., Goodman, H. V. and Vahrman, J.: Gonorrhea with skin and joint manifestations. *Br Med J,* 2:271-274, 1970.
15. Graber, W. J., III, Sanford, J. P. and Ziff, M.: Sex incidence of gonococcal arthritis. *Arthritis Rheum,* 3:309-313, 1960.
16. Wright, V.: Arthritis associated with venereal disease. *Ann Rheum Dis,* 22:77-90, 1963.
17. Keiser, H., Ruben, F. L., Wolinsky, E. and Kushner, I.: Clinical forms of gonococcal arthritis. *N Engl J Med,* 279:234-240, 1968.

18. Holmes, K. K.: Recovery of *Neisseria gonorrhoeae* from sterile synovial fluid in gonococcal arthritis. *N Engl J Med*, 284:318-320, 1971.
19. Bonhoff, M. and Page, M. I.: Experimental infection with parent and L-phase variant of *N. meningitidis. J Bacteriol*, 95:2070-2077, 1968.
20. Fiumura, N. J., Wise, H. M., Jr. and Many, M.: Gonorrheal pharyngitis. *N Engl J Med*, 276:1248-1250, 1967.
21. Metzger, A. L.: Gonococcal arthritis complicating gonorrheal pharyngitis. *Ann Intern Med*, 73:267-269, 1970.
22. Sparling, P. F.: Gonococcal antibiotic resistance. From The VD Crisis. International Venereal Disease Symposium, St. Louis, Mo., 1971.
23. Davis, D. S. and Romansky, M. J.: Successful treatment of gonococcic endocarditis with erythromycin: review of literature. *Am J Med*, 21: 473-479, 1956.
24. Thayer, W. S. and Blumer, G.: Ulcerative endocarditis due to the gonococcus: gonorrheal septicemia. *Bull Hopkins Hosp*, 7:57, 1896.
25. Vietzke, W. M.: Gonococcal arthritis with pericarditis. *Arch Intern Med*, 117:270-272, 1966.
26. Vander Veer, J. B. and Noris, R. F.: The electrocardiographic changes in acute pericarditis. *Am Heart J*, 14:31-50, 1937.
27. Boyle, J. D., Morton, L. P. and Guze, L. B.: Purulent pericarditis: review of literature and report of eleven cases. *Medicine*, 40:119-144, 1961.
28. Shapiro, E., Lipkis, M. L., Kahn, J. and Heid, J. B.: Electrocardiographic changes in acute gonococcal arthritis and myocarditis simulating acute rheumatic polyarthritis. *Am J Med Sci*, 217:300-307, 1949.
29. Curtis, A. H.: A cause of adhesions in the right upper quadrant. *JAMA*, 94:1221-1222, 1930.
30. Fitz-Hugh, T.: Acute gonococcic peritonitis of the right upper quadrant in women. *JAMA*, 102:2094-2096, 1934.
31. Fitz-Hugh, T.: Acute gonococcic perihepatitis: a new syndrome of right upper quadrant abdominal pain in young women. *Rev Gastroent*, 3:125-131, 1936.
32. Kimball, M. W. and Knee, S.: Gonococcal perihepatitis in a male. The Fitz-Hugh-Curtis syndrome. *N Engl J Med*, 1082-1084, 1970.
33. Lichtman, S. S.: Gonococcal endocarditis with jaundice. *J Mount Sinai Hosp NY*, 4:72-76, 1937.
34. Steiner, W. R. and Walton, L. L.: Gonorrheal endocarditis with bilateral parotitis and toxic jaundice as additional complications. *Ann Intern Med*, 11:1464-1471, 1938.
35. Fued, G. L.: Gonococcal peritonitis in a prepubertal child. *Am J Dis Child*, 115:621-622, 1968.
36. Smith, D.: Gonococcal meningitis. *Lancet*, 1:1217, 1922.
37. Bradford, W. L. and Kelley, H. W.: Gonococcic meningitis in a newborn infant. *Am J Dis Child*, 46:543-549, 1933.

38. Stigler, S. L. and McLester, J. S.: Gonococcic meningitis fifteen years after urethritis. *JAMA*, 136:919-920, 1948.

39. Lampe, W. T.: Gonococcal meningitis complicating treated gonococcal urethritis. *Ann Intern Med*, 59:94-96, 1963.

40. Vidal, E.: Eruption generalisee et symetrique de croutes cornees avec chute des ongles d'origine blenorhagrique coincidante avec une polyarthrite de meme nature. *Ann Dermatol Syphiligr* (Paris), 4:3, 1893.

41. Abu-Nassar, H., Hill, N., Fred, H. L. and Yow, E. M.: Cutaneous manifestations of gonococcemia. A review of 14 cases. *Arch Intern Med*, 112:731-737, 1963.

42. Ackerman, A. B., Miller, R. C. and Shapiro, L.: Gonococcemia and its cutaneous manifestations. *Arch Dermatol*, 91:227-232, 1965.

43. Ackerman, A. B.: Hemorrhagic bullae in gonococcemia. *N Engl J Med*, 282:793-794, 1970.

44. Keil, H.: A type of gonococcal bacteremia with characteristic hemorrhagic vesicopustular and bullous lesions. *Q J Med*, 7:1-15, 1938.

45. Kahn, G. and Danielson, D.: Septic gonococcal dermatitis; demonstration of gonococci and gonococcal antigens in skin lesions by immunofluorescence. *Arch Dermatol*, 99:421-425, 1969.

46. Schmidt, H., Hjorting-Hansen, E. and Philipsen, H. P.: Gonococcal stomatitis. *Acta Derm Venereol* (Stockh), 41:324-327, 1961.

47. Copping, N.: Stomatitis caused by gonococcus. *J Am Dent Assoc*, 49: 567, 1954.

48. Diefenbacher, W. C. L.: Gonorrheal parotitis. *Oral Surg*, 6:974-975, 1953.

49. Thatcher, R. W. and Petit, T. H.: Gonorrheal conjunctivitis. *JAMA*, 215:1494-1496, March 1, 1971.

50. Friendly, D. S.: Gonococcal conjunctivitis of the newborn. *Clin Proc Child Hosp DC*, 25:1-5, 1969.

51. Hilton, A. L.: PAM plus probenecid in gonorrhea and procaine penicillin plus probenecid in gonorrhea. *Br J Vener Dis*, 47:107-110, 1971.

52. Van Steenbergen, E. P.: Treatment of gonorrhea with single oral doses. *Br J Vener Dis*, 47:111-113, 1971.

53. Groth, O. and Hallquist, L.: Oral ampicillin in gonorrhea: clinical evaluation. *Br J Vener Dis*, 46:21-26, 1970.

54. Ongom, V. L.: A "single dose" treatment of gonococcal urethritis with rifampicin. *Br J Vener Dis*, 47:188-189, 1971.

55. Willcox, R. R.: A survey of problems in the antibiotic treatment of gonorrhea. *Br J Vener Dis*, 46:217-242, 1970.

56. Cornelius, C. E. and Domescik, G.: Spectinomycin hydrochloride in the treatment of uncomplicated gonorrhea. *Br J Vener Dis*, 46:212-213, 1970.

CHAPTER 10

SYPHILIS IN THE NEGRO

JOHN A. KENNEY, JR.

THE TITLE OF THIS SECTION, *Syphilis in the Negro*—or to use modern-day parlance, *Syphilis in Blacks*—would imply that the disease manifests itself differently in Negroes than it does in whites, that there is something distinctive about the disease in the black, that it is more or less virulent in this racial group or that there are other differences in the behavior of *Treponema pallidum* when it is implanted in blacks as opposed to whites. If there is any *message* to be derived from this brief Chapter and any justification for including it in a work of this kind it is to state that there is some question about this, and we as yet do not have sufficient data to establish a racial difference of this kind as an unequivocal fact. Although a racial difference has been alleged to exist in the past, it is difficult to document, and it appears to have been based on generalizations, opinions and beliefs rather than on statistically verified evidence. Although there are figures showing a higher reported incidence of syphilis in blacks than in whites, causing some to conclude that the disease is more prone to affect blacks, such a belief is open to question. To quote the recent report, *Today's V.D. Control Problem —1972:*

> "Venereal diseases are notoriously under-reported by private physicians, but are nearly completely reported by public clinics. The socioeconomically deprived (of whom nonwhites comprise a disproportionate segment) tend to seek medical care from public clinics and are far more likely to be reported than those treated by private physicians. Consequently, there is considerable bias reflected in the higher reported incidence rate among nonwhites." (1)

Parran (2) wrote that "Wherever education and living conditions among the Negro race approximate that of the white race, the syphilis rate approximates that of the white." Brown and his associates (3) state the situation from a somewhat different perspective, as follows:

> "The differentials in mortality between the white and nonwhite populations are the end-product of a multidimensional problem. Some of the factors that may affect this problem include the distribution and availability of medical facilities and services, socioeconomic factors which affect the utilization of available medical services, and the personal motivation to achieve better health. Further study is needed to determine more accurately the degree that color and sex affect the risk of dying among a group of syphilitics."

Chief among the supposedly distinctive features of syphilis in the Negro is the occurrence of annular secondary syphilis lesions. Hinton (4), a Negro himself, wrote that annular lesions are "more common among Negroes." Thomas (5) stated "Annular lesions superficially resembling ringworm infections are observed almost exclusively in Negroes." Stokes and his associates (6) stated "Annular secondary syphilids occasionally appear upon the face in white patients. They are much more common and of more general distribution in the colored patient." In view of this general agreement among such eminent authorities as the ones cited, one must accept as probable fact that annular lesions are seen more frequently in Negro patients. However, Fiumara (7) has pointed out that he has frequently seen annular lesions in white patients and states it is his belief that annular lesions are largely a reflection of the length of time that the patient has had the disease. He suspects it may well be that blacks generally are slower to come in for treatment than whites—possibly because of the same socioeconomic reasons given by Brown and his associates (3) above—and the disease has thus been given a longer time in which to develop annular lesions.

There also seems to be some agreement among authorities that the pustular syphilid is seen more frequently in Negroes than in whites (8, 9, 10).

Still another often cited racial difference in the behavior of *T. pallidum* in whites and blacks is contained in the following quotation by Kierland (11) in his section on syphilis in the Ormsby-Montgomery textbook, *Diseases of the Skin:*

"The race to which the patient belongs also plays a part in the type of late syphilis, as may be expected. The incidence of neurosyphilis is twice as great in the white race as in the Negro; on the other hand, cardiovascular syphilis is more frequent in the Negro than in the white race."

This statement does appear to be fairly well documented and is widely accepted. A recent author, Friedman (12), found three times as many Negro as white patients with cardiovascular syphilis, which was in distinct contrast to the ratio in the overall hospital population which was one Negro to three white subjects. The same author (13) found that neurosyphilis was more frequent among white subjects than among blacks. He wrote "The racial difference in incidence of neurosyphilis was particularly striking in the symptomatic varieties (tabes, paresis, meningovascular) which occurred more than twice as often in white than in Negro syphilitic cardiacs."

One could continue along this same vein, citing other references from the literature to buttress this or that point with regard to racial differences in the disease as it affects blacks and whites, but one has the feeling that one is *shadow boxing*, that much more documentation is needed with more control over the many variables which seem to affect the statistics, more control over the socioeconomic factors, for example, and the others which bear so heavily on the situation.

One might well conclude with a quotation from Lewis (13) as follows:

"There is a possibility that there is a more basic cause for the racial characteristics of syphilis which is analogous to the suggested cause of the racial differences in tuberculosis. Syphilis, like tuberculosis, is greatly influenced by tissue immunity, which is usually directly acquired but which may also be acquired in some degree by inheritance. Negroes have not been in contact with syphilis as long as have most white races, and there probably has not been the opportunity to develop the same racial resistance through the forces of natural selection."

REFERENCES

1. American Social Health Association: *Today's VD Control Problem—1972.* New York, 1972, p. 18-19.
2. Parran, T.: *Shadow on the Land.* New York, Reynal, 1937, p. 177.

3. Brown, W. J., Donohue, J. F., Axnick, N. W., Blount, J. H., Ewen, N. H. and Jones, O. G.: *Syphilis and Other Venereal Diseases.* Cambridge, Harvard U Pr, 1970, p. 115.

4. Hinton, W. A.: *Syphilis and Its Treatment.* New York, Macmillan, 1936, p. 67.

5. Thomas, E. W.: *Syphilis: Its Course and Management.* New York, Macmillan, 1949, p. 157.

6. Stokes, J. H., Beerman, H. and Ingraham, N. R., Jr.: *Modern Clinical Syphilology,* 3rd ed. Philadelphia, Saunders, 1944, p. 527.

7. Fiumara, N. J.: Personal Communication.

8. Stokes, J. H., Beerman, H. and Ingraham, N. R., Jr., *op. cit.,* p. 531.

9. Hazen, H. H.: *Syphilis.* St. Louis, Mosby, 1919, p. 119.

10. McKenna, C. H., Hahn, R. D. and Cluff, L. E.: Syphilis and other venereal diseases. In Harvey, A. M., Cluff, L. E., Johns, R. J., Owens, A. H., Jr., Rabinowitz, D. and Ross, R. R.: *The Principles and Practice of Medicine,* 17th ed. New York, Appleton, 1968, p. 776.

11. Kierland, R. R.: Syphilis. In Ormsby, O. S. and Montgomery, H.: *Diseases of the Skin,* 8th ed. Philadelphia, Lea and Febiger, 1954, p. 1022.

12. Friedman, B.: Syphilitic aortic insufficiency: some observations on a vanishing disorder. *Ala J Med Sci,* 6:8-17, 1969.

13. Lewis, J. H.: *The Biology of the Negro.* Chicago, U of Chicago Pr, 1942, p. 183.

CHAPTER 11

INTERRELATIONS OF SYPHILIS, YAWS AND PINTA

Rafael Medina

SYPHILIS, YAWS AND PINTA for a long time have been the subject of discussion as to whether three entirely different diseases are involved, or the three are clinical modalities of one and the same affection. Hypotheses have been put forward attributing a common origin to *Treponema pallidum, T. pertenue* and *T. carateum,* saying that ecological factors have, in the course of centuries, modified their way of behaviour within the human organism.

Syphilis still holds its place as a serious public health problem in many countries throughout the world due to the fact that the resources that have been used to combat it have not yielded the expected benefits. This has led to further endeavors to study more basic aspects, which include everything pertaining to its connections and clinical immunological discrepancies with pinta and yaws.

In a summarized form we shall point out the features which draw the three clinical conditions together and the differences which exist among the same.

EPIDEMIOLOGY

Syphilis is predominantly contracted by sexual contact; it is a venereal disease, and its prevalence is in strict relationship with promiscuity and homosexual ratios. Yaws and pinta are rural and sylvan endemias which are only spread by familiar contact, and the incidence manifests decline in all of the world areas where sanitary campaigns have been conducted for its treatment and hygienic conditions have improved. Along these lines, it should be recalled that in certain Afro-Asiatic and tropical American countries yaws has become almost extinct, and pinta, an autochthonous and exclusive treponematosis of the American continent, is being confined progressively to more and more isolated and far-apart areas.

CLINICAL ASPECTS

Differences in clinical manifestations observed in the three treponematoses have served as a basis to regard them as different and separate ailments. Syphilis affects internal organs, especially the cardiovascular and the neuro-ophthalmological systems; the syphilitic pregnant woman may infect the fetus and thus cause congenital syphilis. Yaws attacks only the skin, mucosae, joints and bones, while pinta limits its action to the skin and related tissue. Neither congenital yaws nor congenital pinta have ever been observed. Study of certain organic manifestations reveals, however, some similarities, such as: osteitis and syphilitic mucocutaneous gummas which are clinically indistinguishable from those produced by yaws, the histopathology being identical; pianides, hypochromic, desquamative spots from the secondary period of yaws bear a great resemblance to certain macular pinta lesions and may even be mistaken for certain syphilides. It is also opportune to recall the similarity displayed by superficial adenopathy.

A summary, even in rough outline, of the clinical aspects of pinta and yaws permits better comparison with syphilis.

Yaws

After an average incubation period of from twelve to twenty-five days, the initial lesion is a vegetating ulceration (mother-yaws) that occurs predominantly on exposed areas. In most cases, from two to eight months after initiation of the process, skin ulcerations occur in a variable number. These are of lesser size than the initial ulcer but exhibit the same clinical features; on occasion, the secondary outbreak is dominated by hypochromic desquamative maculae (pianides). Secondary lesions likewise

Sexually Transmitted Diseases

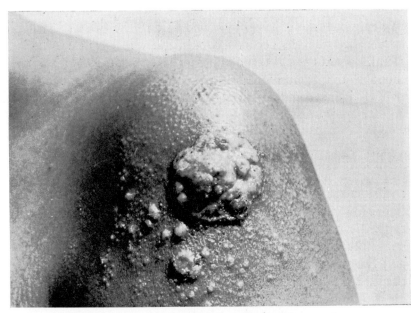

Figure XI-1. Yaws: Primary lesion (mother-yaw).

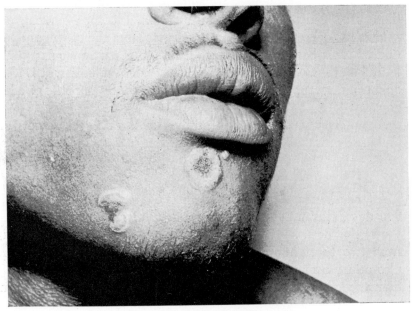

Figure XI-2. Yaws: secondary stage.

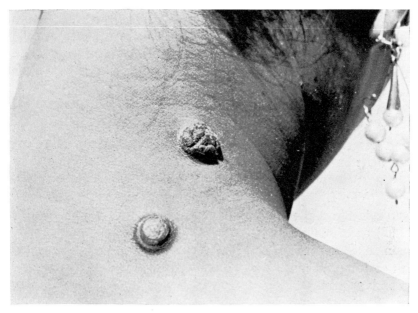

Figure XI-3. Yaws: crusted secondary lesions.

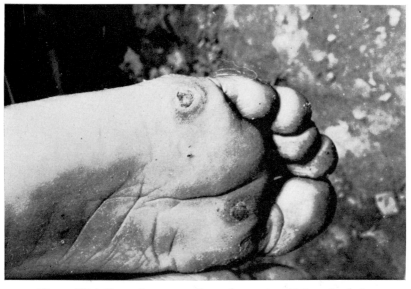

Figure XI-4. Yaws: late stage (hyperkeratotic nodules of soles).

tend to disappear spontaneously, and after, a prolonged or final latent phase of the disease sets in (Figs. XI-2 to XI-3). Late complications consist of cutaneous hyperkeratosis, usually on the plantar surfaces, osteoperiostitis, articular inflammations, mutilating rhinopharyngitis and cutaneous or osseous gummas; these complications may appear either isolated or simultaneously.

From the serological viewpoint, circulating antibodies appear in yaws sufferers within eighteen to thirty days after initiation of the disease. The titers consistently remain high during the first few years but tend to oscillate when the late phase of the disease sets in, such oscillations being more marked in flocculation reactions (VDRL type) and complement fixation tests (Kolmer type), in the majority of yaws sufferers, than in immobilization (TPI) and immunofluorescence (FTA-ABS) reactions which remain indefinitely reactive. The evolution of yaws is completed in two stages. The *early* stage is during which the primary and secondary manifestations appear with a combined average dura-

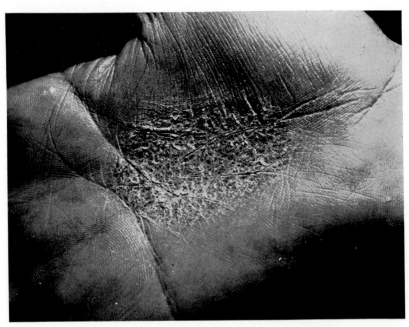

Figure XI-5. Yaws: hyperkeratotis of the palm.

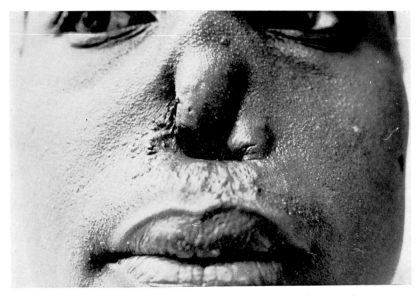

Figure XI-6. Yaws: rhinopharyngitis mutilans (gangosa).

tion of from two to three years. The skin lesions during this phase contain a large number of treponemes, and this is the time when the disease is transmissible. Thereafter, the *late* stage sets in, and it is hardly possible to detect treponemes with the dark-field microscope, in the skin lesions or mucosae. In the great majority of cases, just like in syphilis, clinical alterations appear with a certain orderly fashion in the course of time.

Pinta

The incubation period generally is from ten to thirty-five days, but on occasion it may be of several months. The initial lesion is a flat papule predominantly on cutaneous areas which are more apt to be exposed. It grows slowly and at the end of a few weeks it may appear as an erythematous plaque, slightly infiltrated at the edges and hypochromic in the center. The initial lesion is usually single and tends to disappear spontaneously after a period of a few weeks to one year, or even longer. Whether or not the initial lesion is present, regularly in the intervening period

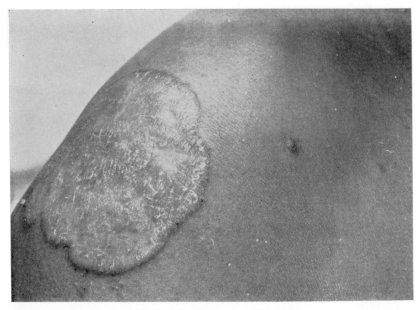

Figure XI-7. Pinta: initial macule.

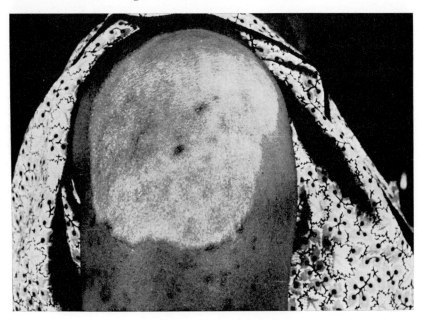

Figure XI-8 Pinta: large initial lesion.

between the third and the eighth months, there appear the so-
called secondary lesions (pintides) which consist of erythematous hypochromic or pigmented maculae in variable number covered by a fine-textured and adherent scale. After the second
year, macular lesions gradually succeed in covering varying sized
areas of the face, trunk and limbs; some become hyperkeratotic,
others undergo atrophy. The nails and hairy regions may be in-
vaded. In the course of years, the macules over prominences,
such as the elbows, knees and ankles, generally turn achromic
(Figs. XI-10 to XI-14). After the first year, generalized superficial
lymphadenopathy is a common occurrence. Pinta is unlike syphilis and yaws where, as we have already mentioned, the lesions
show a rather orderly sequence of evolution, and treponemes are
readily demonstrated in the early skin lesions. In pinta, at any
time during its long, drawn-out evolution, it is common to wit-
ness the appearance of maculae identical with those seen at the
onset, and the demonstration of treponemes is always possible
throughout the course of the disease in any type of lesion, with

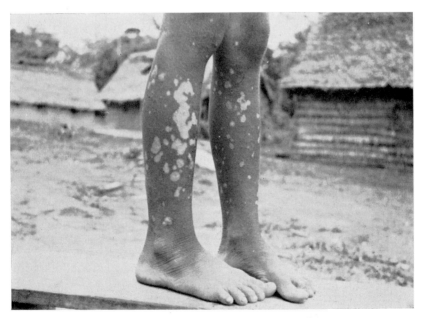

Figure XI-9. Pinta: erythematous secondary lesions.

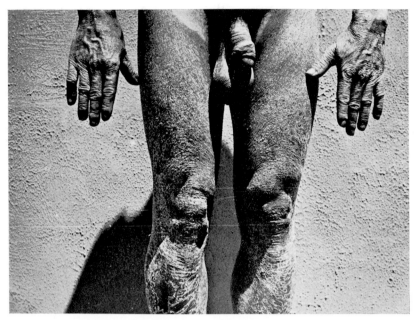

Figure XI-10. Pinta: late phase (extensive pigmentary lesions).

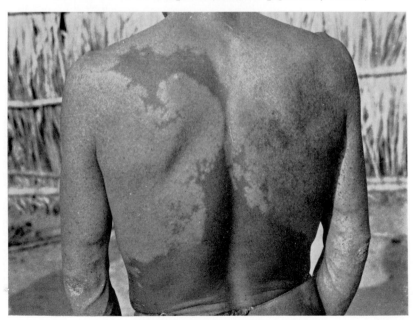

Figure XI-11. Pinta: hypochromic lesions.

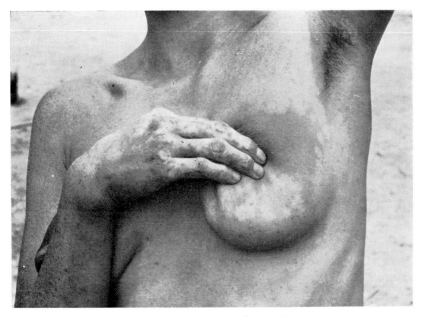

Figure XI-12. Pinta: hypochromic lesions.

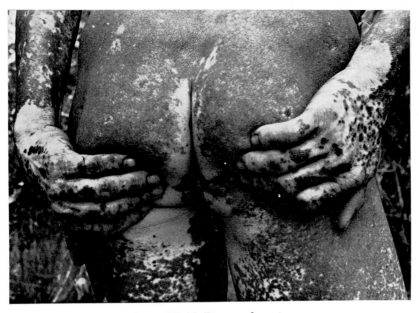

Figure XI-13. Pinta: achromic.

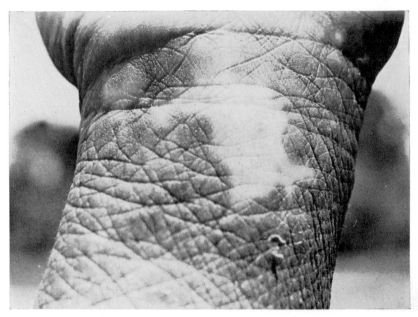

Figure XI-14. Pinta: late atrophy.

the exception of the achromic ones. Pinta is potentially contagious throughout its evolution. Serological antibodies appear between forty-five to ninety days after commencement of the disease. With the cardiolipin antigens, reactivity tends to oscillate, but immunofluorescence remains strongly reactive indefinitely.

Cross Immunology

Comparative immunological study of human treponematoses presents very peculiar and interesting aspects. *Treponema pallidum, T. pertenue* and *T. carateum* determine the formation, in both humans and in certain experimental animals, of circulating antibodies that are absolutely undistinguishable with the resources which are presently available. Insofar as cross immunology of the three diseases is concerned, significant differences are observed. In medical practice in the countries where these diseases are endemic, pinta sufferers, after the second year of evolution, have never been known to have contracted syphilis or yaws.

On the contrary, it is not uncommon to observe the development of pinta in patients who suffer, or have suffered, from yaws in the past. From the experimental point of view, we have been able to prove this partial cross resistance by inoculating a significant number of patients who had pinta of more than two years' duration with *T. pallidum* and *T. pertenue* extracted from human lesions. None of them exhibited signs of infection after being followed for a reasonable time. By contrast, we were able to produce pinta infection by inoculating syphilitic and yaws patients in any stage. In experimental animals, also, the treponemas behave in a different fashion. With *T. pallidum* it has been possible to infect various animals, the rabbit being the prototype; with *T. pertenue*, infection has likewise been produced in animals, of which the hamster appears to be the most selective one; and with *T. carateum* it has been possible to infect only chimpanzee monkeys.

REFERENCES

Guthe, T. and Reynolds, F.: World health and treponematoses. *Br J Vener Dis*, 27:1, 1951.

Itriago, P. M. and Medina, R.: Contribucion al estudio de la buba en Venezuela. *Arch Venez Pat Trop*, 1:193, 1949.

Medina, R.: Pinta, an endemic treponematose of the Americas. *WHO*, 204: 65, 1965.

Simons, R. D. G.: *Handbook of Tropical Dermatology and Medical Mycology*. New York, Am Elsevier, 1952-1953.

Turner, T. B.: Studies on the relationship between yaws and syphilis. *Am J Hyg*, 25:477, 1937.

Turner, T. B. and Chesney, A.: Experimental yaws; 2. Comparison of the infection with experimental syphilis. *Bull Johns Hopkins Hosp*, 54:174, 1934.

CHAPTER 12

VENEREAL HERPES SIMPLEX VIRUS INFECTIONS

André J. Nahmias
William E. Josey
AND
Zuher M. Naib

SINCE THE FIRST DESCRIPTION of genital herpes by Astruc in 1736, physicians with special interest in venereal diseases have recorded many observations contributing to our understanding of the clinical and epidemiological aspects of this disease. In the 19th century such workers detailed the clinical manifestations of genital herpes, observed that the disease was common in prostitutes and in patients attending venereal disease clinics but rare in children and noted that it frequently coexisted with syphilis and gonorrhea. These early venereologists also surmised that genital herpes was in some way related to sexual intercourse, although they did not realize its infectious nature at the time.

The viral cause of genital herpes was established in the first part of this century, soon after Grüter was able to transmit herpes simplex virus to the rabbit cornea. Until recently, the viruses of *herpes febrilis* and that of *venereus herpes* were believed to be identical, even though Lipschütz maintained as early as 1921 that the two viruses were different. The venereal mode of transmission of genital herpes was also doubted by many physicians.

These issues were resolved as a result of studies conducted by our group and others within the past five years. Earlier observations of Schneweis and Plummer, demonstrating the existence of two antigenically different types of herpes simplex virus (HSV-1 and HSV-2), were confirmed and extended to show that HSV-2 is isolated primarily from genital sites and is venereally transmitted, as compared to HSV-1, which is most frequently recovered from nongenital sites and is rarely venereally transmitted.

GENERAL PERSPECTIVE

In placing the clinical and epidemiological aspects of genital herpes in a perspective familiar to the venereologist, it might be useful to point out first the many analogous features of genital herpes and gonorrhea (Tables 12-I and 12-II). Both HSV-2 and *Neisseria gonorrhoeae* have a particular propensity for the genital organs and are primarily transmitted venereally or from the moth-

TABLE 12-I

CLINICAL ASPECTS OF GONOCOCCAL AND GENITAL
HERPES (TYPE 2) INFECTIONS

	Gonorrhea	*Genital Herpes (Type 2)*
I. Involvement of genital organs		
A. Females		
Symptoms	Most often asymptomatic in cervix	Most often asymptomatic in cervix
Sites of infection	Cervix and urethra, rarely vagina, endometrium, Fallopian tubes	Cervix and vulva, rarely vagina, urethra
Hormonal effect	Probable	Probable
Sequelae	Infertility	Abortions?
B. Males		
Symptoms	May be asymptomatic in urethra; dysuria, urethritis, inguinal adenopathy infrequent; may affect prostate and epididymis	May be asymptomatic in urethra; dysuria, urethritis, inguinal adenopathy (primary cases); may affect prostate and epididymis
Complications	Urethral strictures	Urethral strictures (infrequent)
II. Extragenital involvement		
Both sexes	Proctitis, pharyngitis, skin lesions, bacteremia, meningitis, ophthalmia in adult, arthritis, endocarditis, peritonitis	Proctitis, pharyngitis, skin lesions, viremia, meningitis

TABLE 12-II

EPIDEMIOLOGICAL PATTERNS OF GONOCOCCAL AND GENITAL
HERPES (TYPE 2) INFECTIONS

	Gonorrhea	Genital Herpes (Type 2)
Frequency (general)	Low socioeconomic > high socioeconomic, common in VD clinics, common in prostitutes, rare in nuns	Low socioeconomic > high socioeconomic, common in VD clinics, common in prostitutes, rare in nuns
Age	Highest in 15-24 yrs. age group, lower rates after age 50 yrs., infrequent in children	Highest in 15-24 yrs. age group, lower rates after age 50 yrs., infrequent in children
Reservoir	Women, chonic infection and reinfection common	Probably women, recurrences (latency? chronic infection? reinfection?)
Attack rate in contacts	1 in 3 to 1 in 5	About 2 in 3
Transmission to newborn from infected mother	Around time of delivery (neonatal ophthalmia)	Primarily around time of delivery (neonatal herpes)

er's infected genital tract to the infant. They both have very
close microbial relatives, HSV-1 and *Neisseria meningitidis,*
agents which do not ordinarily spread venereally, but which can
be found occasionally in the genitalia. Not only are there many
analogies in the clinical aspects and epidemiological patterns of
gonorrheal and genital herpetic infections, but the two agents
not infrequently can infect an individual at the same time.

CLINICAL MANIFESTATIONS

The cervix is the principal site for type 2 HSV infection in
women. As in gonorrhea, the infection is usually asymptomatic,
and the reservoir is most likely cervically-infected women. Unless
characteristic vesicular and ulcerative lesions are present, it is
often difficult to diagnose herpetic cervicitis clinically. In pregnant women with a primary infection, cervical involvement may
be severe and present as a necrotizing lesion; in such cases, the
virus may be recovered up to three months. Usually, however, the
virus will persist in the cervix for less than a month, but the infection may recur at that site at varying intervals.

Vaginal lesions are infrequent, but when present the vesicles or ulcers are usually confined to the vaginal fornices. Type 2 herpetic vulvitis is unusual in the absence of cervical infection and may precede or follow herpetic cervicitis. The clinical diagnosis of genital herpes in women is most often made by finding single or multiple vesicles and ulcers on the vulva or perineal skin. The lesions occasionally spread to involve the thighs or buttocks.

In the male, the diagnostic vesicles and ulcers are usually found on the glans penis, prepuce or balano-preputial sulcus. The lesions may also occur on the shaft of the penis and less commonly on the scrotum, thighs or buttocks. In both sexes the lesions, unless secondarily infected, heal without scarring.

Type 2 HSV infections occur most commonly in individuals who had experienced HSV-1 infections during childhood. An HSV-2 infection occurring in an individual with no prior HSV-1 or HSV-2 antibodies (primary infection) is usually more severe than if either HSV-1 and/or HSV-2 antibodies are already present. Such primary infections are often accompanied by fever, regional lymphadenopathy and constitutional symptoms. As a result of homosexual or oral-genital contact, type 2 HSV can also cause perianal or oral lesions.

Genital herpes in either sex can be associated with urethral involvement and dysuria, and in severe cases may even cause urinary retention. It has also been shown that males may carry HSV asymptomatically in the urethra, prostate and vas deferens. The fact that herpetic urethritis can occur in the absence of other lesions suggests that HSV infection may account for some cases of *nonspecific urethritis*. Herpetic cystitis and prostatitis have also been described. In view of all the urogenital sites, other than the external genitalia, which can be involved by herpes simplex virus, we suggest that the term *herpes progenitalis* is no longer very meaningful and should be abandoned.

As with type 1 HSV infection (e.g. cold sores), type 2 HSV infections also tend to recur in many individuals. It is not clear at present whether some of the genital recurrences could be a result of exogenous reinfection. This source of recurrent virus would be unlikely to explain the repeated bouts of infection known to occur in some women around the time of their menstrual period.

Recurrent lesions on the external genitalia are often closely ar-
ranged in groups and may go unnoticed by the patient. In some
cases, however, the recurrences may cause severe distress if they
are accompanied by neuralgic pains. Recurrent herpetic cervicitis
is virtually asymptomatic and is most often detected by means
of Papanicolaou cervical smears obtained for routine cervical
cancer screening, which reveal typical cytologic changes of herpetic infection (see Laboratory Diagnosis).

Immediate complications of genital HSV infection are relatively infrequent but may include urethral stricture, secondary
bacterial infection and lymphatic suppuration. More serious,
but apparently usually self-limited complications are meningitis,
radiculitis and ascending myelitis. Genital herpes has also been
associated with some cases of erythema multiforme and may be
responsible for Kaposi's varicelliform eruption in patients with
certain underlying dermatoses, such as atopic dermatitis.

The differential diagnosis of genital herpes includes several
conditions affecting the urogenital organs, particularly other venereal infections. One of the most common misdiagnoses is
chancroid, especially in venereal disease clinics and in military
personnel. Syphilitic chancres, and the early lesions of lymphogranuloma venereum and granuloma inguinale, have also been
confused with genital herpes. Herpetic urethritis and cervicitis
can also be clinically mistaken for gonorrheal infection.

The more prominent primary cervical lesions may raise a clinical suspicion of carcinoma. Other diseases to be differentiated
include herpes zoster, Vincent's infection, Behcet's syndrome,
molluscum contagiosum, erythema multiforme, aberrant vaccin-
ia, impetigo and other dermatoses involving the genitalia.

EPIDEMIOLOGICAL PATTERNS

Since type 2 genital herpes, like gonorrhea, is frequently sub-
clinical, accurate data on the incidence of active infections
(both initial and recurrent) are difficult to obtain. Moreover, as
noted above, genital herpes may be clinically confused with other diseases, so that laboratory confirmation is necessary. The occurrence of genital herpes has been found to vary in different
population groups, depending primarily upon the extent of sex-

ual promiscuity of that group. However, it appears that genital herpes, along with other venereal diseases, is becoming more common nowadays in all socioeconomic levels.

In the absence of national reporting of genital herpes, the only way of gaining some appreciation of its frequency is to compare the number of cases of genital herpes to the number of cases of a reportable venereal disease, like gonorrhea. Such comparative studies performed in women attending venereal disease clinics in England, Sweden and the U.S. indicate that one case of genital herpes could be detected for every five to fourteen cases of gonorrhea. Comparison of the prevalence rates of gonorrhea or genital herpes in other populations of women, such as in hospital private or public clinics, or in family planning clinics, yields a similar ratio. Based on these comparative data and the yearly estimate by the Center for Disease Control of 800,000 cases of gonorrhea occurring in U.S. women, it might be estimated that there are also 60,000 to 160,000 cases of genital herpes. It is probable that the number of cases of genital herpes in males is in the same range.

The estimated yearly number of cases of genital herpes in the U.S. is higher than that for primary and secondary syphilis. Further evidence indicating that genital herpes is a more frequent infection than syphilis is the comparative prevalence of syphilis antibodies and HSV-2 antibodies in different population groups. In lower socioeconomic adolescents, for instance, the frequency of HSV-2 antibodies is 10 to 25 percent and rises to 35 to 60 percent by late adulthood. In higher socioeconomic groups, the frequency of HSV-2 antibodies in adults is around 5 to 10 percent. These rates of HSV-2 antibodies are several times higher than the rates of syphilis antibodies in similar population groups. HSV-2 antibodies are rarely found in the serum of children or nuns and are very often found in the serum of prostitutes.

Prevalence studies, utilizing clinical, virological or cytological methods of detection, again demonstrate differences in the frequency of genital herpes dependent on the type of population studied. For instance, the venereal disease clinic has provided the highest frequency of genital herpes, no matter which method of detection is used. On clinical grounds only, realizing the possibility of misdiagnosis referred to above, it is of interest that as early as 1883, Unna diagnosed genital herpes in 7.6 percent of women and 0.6 percent of men attending venereal disease clinics in Hamburg. In 1967, we obtained similar rates in a VD clinic in Atlanta. Swedish workers have noted more recently a higher percentage (3.8 percent) of men with clinical and virologically-confirmed genital herpes. Virological studies in American or European VD clinics have demonstrated that the frequency of asymptomatic genital herpes in women is between 1.6 percent to 6 percent, and in men is around 1 percent. When cytological methods were employed, the frequency of detection of genital herpes in women was around 3 percent.

The proportion of viral isolation of genital HSV in asymptomatic women studied in hospital clinics has ranged as high as 1.6 percent, and in one cervical cancer detection clinic was found to be 0.1 percent. By the use of Papanicolaou cervical smears to detect the cytological changes associated with herpetic infection in asymptomatic women, the prevalence varied according to the study population. The rate has ranged from 0.02 percent in hospital private clinic patients, to 0.1 percent in planned parenthood clinics, to 0.3 to 0.5 percent of hospital public clinic patients. Two studies done in hospital public clinic women indicated that the frequency of cytologically detected cases of genital herpes was three times greater in pregnant than in nonpregnant women. This observation may reflect the longer duration of viral persistence during pregnancy or an influence of pregnancy on herpetic recurrences. It is of interest, in this regard, that pregnancy also increases the rate of recovery of cytomegalovirus from the cervix.

As with gonorrhea, genital herpes is more prevalent among teenagers and young adults. Teenagers were found in one study to constitute one half of females with virologically or cytologically detected infection and one fourth of males with virologically confirmed infection. Several other studies have detected genital herpes most frequently in individuals below the age of twenty-five years. Serologic studies have further shown that patients with evidence of primary type 2 HSV infection, i.e. with neither HSV-1 or HSV-2 antibodies in the acute phase serum, had a mean age of eighteen and a median age of nineteen years.

Genital herpes is not uncommonly found to coexist with other genital infections. For instance, three studies in VD clinics suggest that one out of every ten to twenty women infected with gonorrhea will have a concomitant genital herpetic infection. Other infections also seen together with genital herpes include syphilis, trichomoniasis, venereal warts, pediculosis pubis and inclusion vaginitis (TRIC agent). Examples of coexisting genital infections, observed by us, include the concomitant detection of type 2 herpetic cervicitis and urethritis, gonococcal cervicitis and condylomata of the vulva and vagina in a woman, and coexisting gonococcal pharyngitis and HSV-2 oral infection in a man.

All of the above observations are quite consistent with the patterns of a venereal disease. The best support for venereal transmission are two contact studies of males with penile herpes. Both investigations demonstrate that at least two thirds of the female contacts showed evidence of active genital herpes. Experimental support for the venereal mode of transmission has also been obtained by the demonstration that male mice or rabbits developed penile herpes when exposed to genitally HSV-infected female mice or rabbits. At least two other herpesviruses of animals, one affecting cows and one horses, are also venereally transmitted.

A note of caution needs to be introduced here as regards attributing all genital herpetic infections to some form of venereal contact. About 5 percent of genital herpetic infections in males or females have been found to be due to HSV-1. The origin of the herpesvirus in some of these cases has been observed to be auto-infection from a concomitant oral type 1 infection. The finding of type 1 penile herpes and type 1 vulvar and oral herpes in a husband-wife couple suggests that on occasion HSV-1 can be transmitted by some form of venereal contact. It should also be pointed out that, as with syphilis and gonorrhea, some HSV-2 infections may be transmitted by means other than sexual contact. We have observed, for instance, a family of a husband, wife and daughter with HSV-2 infection of the buttocks in whom transmission might have resulted from toilet-seat contact. The isolation of HSV-2 from the hand of a nun working in a hospital and of a technician working with the virus, also demonstrates the occasional nonsexual acquisition of HSV-2.

LABORATORY DIAGNOSIS

The virological confirmation of HSV infection has been facilitated recently by the availability of a transport medium which allows shipment of clinical specimens at ambient temperature to virology laboratories in health departments or other institutions. The virus can be demonstrated in various tissue cultures usually within one to three days. Further typing of HSV isolates can now be performed readily by several serological methods. In addition, it is possible to identify and type directly HSV from clinical specimens by immunofluorescent techniques.

Cytological or histological demonstration of multinucleated giant cells and intranuclear inclusions is also a rapid way to detect an HSV infection. In the large majority of cases, varicella and herpes zoster which produce similar cellular changes can be differentiated on clinical grounds. Exfoliative cytology of cervicovaginal smears has been particularly useful in the detection of asymptomatic genital herpetic infections in women.

Although complement fixation tests help occasionally in demonstrating a primary infection, more finite serological tests are required to differentiate HSV type antibodies. At present, such tests are only available in specialized laboratories and lack complete specificity in differentiating the two types of HSV antibodies. It is also possible now to demonstrate HSV antibodies in specific IgG, IgA or IgM serum fractions. A model in Cebus monkeys for the study of genital herpes, which mimics closely observations made in humans, has also recently been developed.

PREVENTION AND TREATMENT

There are no definitive measures now known to prevent genital herpes infection. The effectiveness of condoms for this purpose has not been evaluated. Since it is not known at present if males with penile herpes can carry the virus asymptomatically in the urethra between recurrences, it is unclear whether the use of a condom or sexual abstention when a male has active penile lesions would be sufficient to prevent transmission to his female contact. However, such methods might be recommended to infected male contacts of pregnant women, particularly in the last trimester. We have noted, for instance, the spread of virus from a male with recurrent penile herpes to his pregnant wife late in pregnancy who, after developing a primary genital infection, transmitted HSV-2 to her newborn; the infant then succumbed from a disseminated herpetic infection. A possible approach for preventing genital spread of the virus from a pregnant woman around the time of delivery to her newborn is performance of cesarean section prior to rupture of membranes. This procedure needs to be individualized, as the evidence for its effectiveness is still not definitive.

The treatment of genital herpes is at present largely symptomatic. The main considerations are relief of discomfort and prevention of secondary bacterial infection in lesions on the external genitalia. The rare instances of secondary infection may be treated with topical antibacterial ointments. Topical preparations containing corticosteroids are considered to be contraindicated.

None of the various therapeutic measures which have been recommended over the years for treating recurrent herpes simplex lesions have been shown to be reliably curative. The use of smallpox vaccinations is not recommended on account of its lack of efficacy in controlled studies and the potential complications which may result in certain immunosuppressed patients. An experimental type 1 herpesvirus vaccine, produced by Eli Lilly and Co., may have value in treating recurrent type 1 infections, but appears to be ineffective against type 2 recurrent infection. A type 2 herpesvirus vaccine has been used in West Germany but is not available in the U.S.

Results with topical iododeoxyuridine (IDU), which is beneficial in treating herpetic keratitis, have not, in general, been found to be very helpful in the treatment of genital herpes. A method of treatment using a special dye in conjunction with fluorescent light has recently been reported, but is too new for evaluation of long-term results.

LONG-TERM IMPLICATIONS OF GENITAL HERPES

In its long-term implications to health, genital herpes bears some resemblance to syphilis, particularly if one were at the same point in history when syphilis was only associated with an evanescent sore and rash. Genital herpes usually exhibits several *sores,* and to the afflicted may be most bothersome when it recurs, particularly if the recurrence is also accompanied by neuralgias. However, there is one severe complication of syphilis which is also common to genital herpes—the possible damaging effect on the fetus or newborn. It has been suggested that there is an increased abortion and prematurity rate in infants born to mothers with genital herpetic infection, and that transplacental transmission of HSV can occur. However, more conclusively established is the likelihood for an infant to acquire a herpetic infection if delivered vaginally from a woman with genital herpes around the time of delivery. If the membranes are ruptured prior to cesarean section, the infant is also at risk. The infected newborn may exhibit disseminated disease with a high fatality rate; encephalitis with a significant fatality rate or neurological sequelae in survivors; or ocular involvement with occasional blindness. Even if the infection appears to be localized to the skin of the infant, later evidence of neurological damage may be noted. Many of the clinical manifestations of neonatal herpes resemble those found with syphilis, as well as with toxoplasmosis, rubella, cytomegalovirus and some other infectious agents, such as listeriosis. This complex of perinatal infections, which has so many features in common that a clinical diagnosis cannot most often be made without laboratory aids, has been termed the TORCH group of agents (*T*oxoplasmosis, *O*ther, *R*ubella, *C*ytomegalovirus, *H*erpes simplex virus).

The other presently well-known, long-term implication of syphilis is its involvement of the cardiovascular and neurological systems. The long-term effects of genital herpes are only suggestive at present and are the subject of active current research. Although chronic neurological involvement associated with HSV-2 has been suggested, more studies have been directed toward defining the association noted between genital herpes and cervical neoplasia. It is still unclear to date whether the herpesvirus is causally related to the cervical neoplasia or whether both genital herpes and cervical cancer, acting as venereal diseases, may be coincident in the same woman. In any case, it appears at present that the detection of genital herpes in a woman should serve as an index to obtain careful follow-up for cervical cancer. It might also be noted in this relation that the venereal disease clinic should serve as a focal area for the detection of cervical neoplasia.

ENVOI

Genital herpes has been compared here with gonorrhea, with which it bears many similar clinical and epidemiological features, and with syphilis because of its frequent deleterious effect on the newborn and its possible long-term effects. Present evidence indicates that genital herpes is the second most common venereal disease after gonorrhea, with which it is often detected concomitantly in the same individual. In view of these observations, it is strongly recommended that genital herpes become a reportable venereal disease.

REFERENCES

1. Diday, P. and Doyon, A.: *Les Herpès Génitaux.* Paris, 1886, Masson et Cie.
2. Unna, P. G.: On herpes progenitalis, especially in women. *J Cutan Vener Dis,* 1:321, 1883.
3. Lipschütz, B.: Krankheiten der Herpesgruppe. In Jadassohn, J.: *Handbuch der Haut und Geschlechtskrankheiten.* Berlin, 1932, Springer-Verlag.
4. Nahmias, A. J. and Dowdle, W. R.: Antigenic and biologic differences in *herpesvirus hominis. Progr Med Virol,* 10:110, 1968.
5. Hutfield, D. C.: Herpes genitalis. *Br J Vener Dis,* 44:1, 1968.
6. Josey, W. E., Nahmias, A. J. and Naib, Z. M.: Genital infection with type 2 *herpesvirus hominis:* present knowledge and possible relation to cervical cancer. *Am J Obstet Gynecol,* 101:718, 1968.
7. Yen, S. S. C., Reagan, J. W. and Rosenthal, M. S.: Herpes simplex infection in female genital tract. *Obstet Gynecol,* 25:479-492, 1965.
8. Nahmias, A. J., Dowdle, W. R., Naib, Z. M., Josey, W. E. and Luce, C. F.: Genital infection with *herpesvirus hominis* types 1 and 2 in children. *Pediatrics,* 42:659, 1968.

9. Beilby, J. O. W., Cameron, C. H., Catterall, R. D. and Davidson, D.: *Herpesvirus hominis* infection of the cervix associated with gonorrhea. *Lancet*, 1:1065-1066 (May 18) 1968.
10. Nahmias, A. J., Dowdle, W. R., Naib, Z. M., Josey, W. E., McLone, D. and Domescik, G.: Genital infection with type 2 *herpesvirus hominis*—a commonly occurring venereal disease. *Br J Vener Dis*, 45: 294, 1969.
11. Jeansson, S. and Molin, L.: Genital herpes simplex virus infection. *Lakartidningen*, 68:467, 1971.
12. Rawls, W. E., Gardner, H. L., Flanders, R. W., Lowry, S. P., Kaufman, R. H. and Melnick, J. L.: Genital herpes in two social groups. *Am J Obstet Gynecol*, 110:682, 1971.
13. Nahmias, A. J., Chiang, W., delBuono, I. and Duffey, C.: Typing of *herpesvirus hominis* strains by a direct immunofluorescent technique. *Proc Soc Exper Biol Med*, 132:386, 1969.
14. Rawls, W. E., Tompkins, W. A. F. and Melnick. J. L.: The association of herpesvirus type 2 and carcinoma of the uterine cervix. *Am J Epidemiol*, 89:547, 1969.
15. Nahmias, A. J., Josey, W. E., Naib, Z. M., Luce, C. and Duffey, C.: Antibodies to *herpesvirus hominis* types 1 and 2 in humans. I. Patients with genital herpetic infections. *Am J Epidemiol*, 91:539, 1970.
16. Naib, Z. M., Nahmias, A. J. and Josey, W. D.: Cytology and histopathology of cervical herpes simplex infection. *Cancer*, 19:1026, 1966.
17. Nahmias, A., Wickliffe, C., Pipkin, J., Leibovitz, A. and Hutton, R.: Transport media for herpes simplex viruses types 1 and 2. *Appl Microbiol*, 22:451, 1971.
18. Nahmias, A., delBuono, I., Pipkin, J., Hutton, R. and Wickliffe, C.: Rapid identification and typing of herpes simplex virus types 1 and 2 by a direct immunofluorescence technique. *Appl Microbiol*, 22: 455, 1971.
19. London, W. T., Catalano, L. W., Nahmias, A. J., Fuccillo, D. A. and Sever, J. L.: Genital herpesvirus type 2 infection of monkeys. *Obstet Gynec*, 37:501, 1971.
20. Nahmias, A. J., Alford, C. A. and Korones, S. B.: Infection of the newborn with *herpesvirus hominis*. *Adv Pediatr*, 17:185, 1970.
21. Nahmias, A. J., Josey, W. E., Naib, Z. M., Freeman, M. G., Fernandez, R. J. and Wheeler, J. H.: Perinatal risk associated with maternal genital herpes simplex virus infection. *Am J Obstet Gynecol*, 110: 825, 1971.
22. Nahmias, A., Naib, Z. and Josey, W.: Genital herpes and cervical cancer—can a causal association be proven? In Oncogenesis and Herpesviruses, Biggs, P. M., de Thé, G. and Payne, L. N. (eds). International Agency on Cancer, pp. 403-408, 1972, Lyon.

23. Nahmias, A. J.: Herpesviruses from fish to man—a search for patho-
    biological unity. *Pathobiology Annual*, 2: 1972.
24. Centifanto, Y. M., Drylie, D. M., Deardourff, S. L. and Kaufman,
    H. E.: Herpesvirus type 2 in the male genito-urinary tract. Science
    (in press).

Supported by grants from the Center for Disease Control and the
National Foundation.

CHAPTER 13

LEVELS OF THE SERUM IMMUNOGLOBULINS IgA, IgG AND IgM IN TREATED AND UNTREATED LYMPHOGRANULOMA VENEREUM

A. LASSUS

C. E. SONCK

O. WAGER

AND

K. K. MUSTAKALLIO

LYMPHOGRANULOMA venereum (LGV), the *fourth venereal disease*, is caused by a member of the Chlamydia group of microorganisms. In its subacute form the disease predominantly involves the inguinal and iliacal lymph nodes. When spread through the lymphatics to perirectal tissue, the disease may become quite chronic, causing severe suppurative destruction and stenosis, especially of the rectum.

Patients with LGV often present high levels of serum globulins (Williams and Gutman; Waldenström and others). In a previous study (Lassus and others) we found that as many as six out of eight patients with LGV had elevated levels of at least one of the three immunoglobulins IgA, IgG and IgM. The most consistent finding was the elevation of IgA which occurred in six cases. This finding prompted us to study a larger series.

From 1936 to 1951 one of us (Sonck) examined and treated a large series of patients with LGV in different stages. A number of these patients were traced and called for reexamination. The patients still available were thoroughly examined for activity of the disease, and the level of immunoglobulins was determined. In addition to these old cases, we were able to include a number of new cases with an active disease.

MATERIAL

The series studied included 50 patients with treated or untreated LGV. Ten of the patients, all men who were untreated and had inguinal buboes, had contracted the disease within half a year before the present examination. The mean age of this group was 28 years (range 20 to 37 years). The Frei test was positive in all cases. One of the ten patients had earlier had syphilis (Table 13-I). All ten had been hospitalized at the Department of Dermatology and Venereology, University Central Hospital, Helsinki in 1966 to 1971.

The remaining 40 patients, with a mean age of 37 years (range 24 to 45 years), had an old infection which had been contracted over 20 years before the present study. Thirty-eight of these belonged to the series of Sonck, while two had been lately hospitalized because of active intestinal LGV. Thirty-six of these 40 patients were women. The mean age was 63 years (range 47 to 71 years). All 38 patients of the series of Sonck had had a positive Frei test when tested with a human antigen twelve to forty years before the present study. Thirty-one of these 38,

TABLE 13-I

CLINICAL DATA OF 50 PATIENTS WITH
LYMPHOGRANULOMA VENEREUM

	Acute	Chronic
Total	10	40
Males	10	4
Females		36
Mean age	28 yrs.	63 yrs.
Disease active	10	3
Mean length of time between the first symptoms and the present examination	6 mos.	37 yrs.
Earlier treated with sulphonamides		30
Length of follow-up period in treated cases		28 yrs.
Frei-positive in present study	10	22/33
Syphilis by history	1	10

TABLE 13-II

SEVERITY OF LYMPHOGRANULOMA VENEREUM

	Acute	Chronic
Total	10	40
Ulcers and/or buboes only	10	9
Mild proctitis		7
Intermediate proctitis		5
Severe proctitis		19*

* Seven of these patients had a colostomy.

together with the new patients, were tested with a human Frei antigen (Sonck) in the present examination. Both the new patients and 20 of the 31 earlier-tested patients showed a positive skin reaction with this antigen. Seven of the eleven patients, in which the Frei test had turned negative, either had no intestinal involvement or had suffered only from mild or intermediate proctitis.

Nine of the patients with an old infection had never shown any intestinal involvement, but only a chronic ulcer and/or buboes. Seven of the remaining 31 patients had displayed only a mild proctitis with infiltration but no stenosis or fistulation. In five cases the proctitis had been more severe with stenoses in all cases, but the disease had not been highly destructive. In the remaining nineteen cases the disease had been highly destructive with fistulas and/or stenoses, and in seven of these a colostomy had been performed (Table 13-II). Both the new cases with a chronic infection had severe proctitis. Ten of the 40 patients with an old infection were by history known to have had syphilis (Table I).

METHODS

All the patients were thoroughly examined for activity of the disease. The patients with an old infection were especially examined for an eventual active process in the rectum. In a suspected case a biopsy was taken from the rectal mucosa.

The sera of all patients were examined for syphilitic antilipoidal antibodies with the VDRL slide and Kolmer tests (Lassus) and for treponemal antibodies with the Fluorescent Treponemal Antibody-Absorption (FTA-ABS) test (Lassus).

The serum level of immunoglobulins was in all cases determined by a modification of the single radial immunodiffusion method of Mancini and others. The normal values for the different immunoglobulins with this method as expressed in mg/100 ml serum were: IgA 150 to 520, IgG 800 to 1900, and IgM 30 to 140 (Räsänen and Wager).

RESULTS

None of the ten patients with an infection of short duration had rectal involvement. One of these patients, who was known to have had syphilis, had a serum reactive in the VDRL slide, Kolmer and FTA-ABS tests (Table 13-III). Another patient had a transient reaction in the Kolmer test. This reaction was considered nonspecific since his serum was nonreactive in the FTA-ABS test. The results of the quantitation of the immunoglobulins are presented in the Figures. An elevated level of IgA was found in seven of the ten cases, the mean value being 606 mg/100 ml. Four patients had a slightly elevated level of IgG, mean 1599 mg/100 ml. Two patients had an elevated level of serum IgM, mean 121 mg per 100 ml.

One of the 38 patients of Sonck's series still had an active disease. This was a sixty-two year old man who had contracted LGV at the age of nineteen and had developed suppurating buboes. At the age of twenty-eight he had suffered from a severe proctitis, and the Frei test had been positive. A few years earlier he

TABLE 13-III

TESTS FOR SYPHILIS IN 50 PATIENTS WITH
LYMPHOGRANULOMA VENEREUM

| | Number With Positive Test Results | | |
Tests for Syphilis	Acute	Chronic	Total
VDRL slide	1	1	2
Kolmer	2	1*	3
FTA-ABS	1	11	12

* The sera of three patients were anticomplementary in the Kolmer test.

had contracted syphilis. At the age of thirty he had received sulphonamide treatment (68 gm in all), with some improvement.
However, when reexamined in 1970 he was found to still have
sclerosing infiltrations and fistulas in the anal region, and a biopsy revealed a granulomatotic process in the rectal mucosa. He
still had a positive Frei test. Two women who did not belong to
the series of Sonck had an old active infection. Both had stenoses and fistulas and a positive Frei test. Thus altogether, three of
the present chronic cases had an active disease. The man who was
known to have had syphilis had a serum reactive in the FTA-
ABS test but nonreactive in the antilipoidal tests. The sera of
both women, who by history had not had syphilis, were nonreactive in the VDRL slide and the FTA-ABS test but were anticomplementary in the Kolmer test. Two of the three patients had an
elevated serum level of IgA (Fig. XIII-1). Both women had a

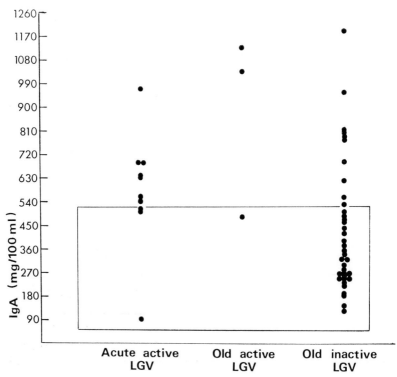

Figure XIII-1. Serum levels of immunoglobulin A in active and inactive
lymphogranuloma venereum (normal range 150 to 520 mg/100 ml serum).

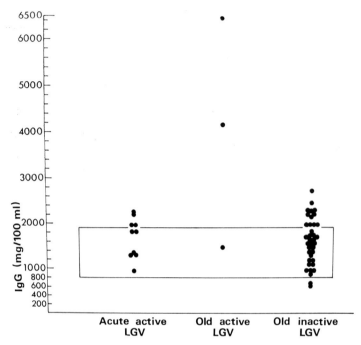

Figure XIII-2. Serum levels of immunoglobulin G in active and inactive lymphogranuloma venereum (normal range 800 to 1900 mg/100 ml serum).

very high level of serum IgG (Fig. XIII-2), while one of the women had an elevated serum level of IgM.

Thirty-seven of the patients with an old infection were regarded as cured. Nine of these were by history known to have had syphilis, and eight of them had serum reactivity in the FTA-ABS test. The sera of two additional patients also proved reactive in the FTA-ABS test despite a negative history of syphilis. Thus altogether, eleven of the thirty-seven patients with an old inactive LGV were regarded to have had syphilis. Only one patient showed serum reactivity in the VDRL slide and Kolmer tests, while the serum of another patient was anticomplementary in the Kolmer test. The latter was one of the two FTA-ABS positive patients without a history of syphilis. She had a normal serum level of immunoglobulins but had both cryoglobulin and rheumatoid factor activity (Waaler-Rose + 128; latex fixation +) in her serum. As illustrated in Table 13-IV, the patients

TABLE 13-IV

LEVELS OF IMMUNOGLOBULINS IN PATIENTS WITH INACTIVE
(CURED) LYMPHOGRANULOMA VENEREUM IN REGARD TO
THE FORMER SEVERITY OF PROCTITIS

Degree of Proctitis	Total No. of Patients	Mean Value of Immunoglobulins (mg/100 ml)		
		IgA	IgG	IgM
No proctitis	9	354	1,483	56
Mild proctitis	7	404	1,411	52
Intermediate proctitis ...	5	372	1,596	87
Severe proctitis	16	451	1,785	54

with severe proctitis seemed to have a somewhat higher serum
level of IgA and IgG than those patients with a milder intestinal
involvement, even after the disease was regarded cured. Altogether ten of the thirty-seven patients had an elevated serum
level of IgA (Fig. XIII-1), mean 413 mg/100 ml serum; five of
these ten had both LGV and syphilis. Eleven patients had an elevated serum level of IgG (Fig. XIII-2), mean 1613 mg/100 ml

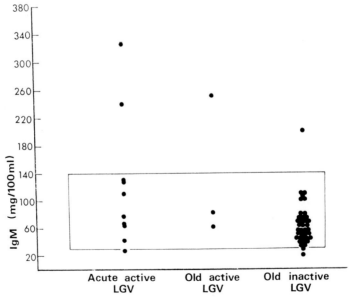

Figure XIII-3. Serum levels of immunoglobulin M in active and inactive
lymphogranuloma venereum (normal range 30-140 mg/100 ml serum).

serum. Five of these were syphilitics. One of these thirty-seven patients had an elevated level of IgM and one a subnormal level of this immunoglobulin.

In the whole series of fifty patients, thirteen (26 percent) had anamnestic or serologic evidence of syphilis. Seven of these had an elevated serum level of IgA (mean 613 mg/100 ml), six an elevated level of IgG (mean 1896 mg/100 ml), while none had an elevated serum level of IgM. One of the thirteen patients had a subnormal level of IgM.

DISCUSSION

Lymphogranuloma venereum is one of the infectious diseases in which prognosis has changed greatly after the introduction of sulphonamide therapy. Before the sulphonamides there was no real treatment for the disease. The sulphonamides and also the later broad-spectrum antibiotics have proven highly effective in preventing later complications of LGV.

LGV, like some other chronic infections, e.g. leprosy, may manifest clinical signs of autoimmune disease such as polyarthritis and erythema nodosum. The infection spreads predominantly through the lymphatics, especially the inguinal and rectal lymph nodes, and may end up as an invasive, destructive process in the intestine. The invasion of the lymphatic system explains the massive immunologic response caused by LGV. Already in 1936 Williams and Gutman described high protein levels of sera in patients with LGV. This was confirmed by Jersild in 1937 in a series of fifty-five LGV-patients. In 1941 Sonck analyzed the serum proteins in 109 LGV-patients, and he found high serum globulin values in most of the active cases of his series. In cured cases the serum protein values were found to be normal.

The quantitation of immunoglobulins in the present study shows some interesting patterns. Only two of the patients with an acute infection showed an elevated level of IgM, four an elevation of IgG and as many as seven of the ten cases an elevation of IgA. The usual immunological response to a fresh infection is a raise of IgM followed by a raise of IgG. This is the case also in the early stages of syphilis. In primary syphilis there is a raised level of IgM, and in secondary syphilis a raised level

of both IgM and IgG (Onisk). According to Delhanty and Catterall, also the level of IgA is often elevated in secondary syphilis. Only one of our patients with an acute LGV had earlier had
syphilis. Therefore, the IgA response of these patients must
have been due to the LGV infection. Recently it has been demonstrated that IgA appears to be the predominant immunoglobulin class in normal seminal fluid (Tomasi and Bienenstock).
This could also be the case for other secretions of the male genital
tract and in part explain the IgA response in acute LGV.

Two of the three patients with a late active LGV also showed
an elevated serum level of IgA. The IgA elevation seems to be
especially connected with the activity of LGV, since over two
thirds of the thirteen patients with an active disease showed such
an elevation.

Two of the three patients with late active LGV had high
levels of IgG, and both had an anticomplementary activity in
the serum. Also, one of the patients with an old inactive LGV
had anticomplementary serum activity despite a normal level of
immunoglobulins, but she had both cryoglobulins and rheumatoid factor activity in her serum. Anticomplementary serum activity indicates the presence of aggregated gammaglobulins,
which may be mere aggregates produced by serum inactivation
or represent circulating immune complexes (Castanedo and Williams) such as a rheumatoid factor or cryoglobulins, which have
been found to be associated with anticomplementary activity
(Lassus and Mustakallio).

One of the patients with old active LGV had an elevated serum level of IgM. This woman had high levels of all three
immunoglobulins.

Over one fourth of the patients with a presumably inactive,
old LGV had elevated serum levels of IgA. One half of these
patients also had syphilis. However, according to Laurell and
others IgA is not elevated in treated syphilis. It therefore seems
that the combination of two chronic diseases might cause an elevated IgA or that these ten patients still might have had an active LGV despite the negative clinical findings. An elevated serum level of IgA might be an indicator for further treatment
of LGV. About one third of the patients with presumably inac-

tive LGV had slightly elevated serum levels of IgG, and one had an elevated IgM. The serum levels of both IgA and IgG seemed to be higher in the cases with a formerly severe, intestinal involvement.

It is of interest that in lepromatous leprosy, which for good reason is regarded as an immune complex disease (Wager 1969), both IgG and IgA are elevated while IgM is normal (Sheagren and others; Wager). Our findings indicate this is the case, also, in most cases of LGV in which there are alterations in the serum immunoglobulins. Increased levels of IgG occur in many longstanding infections, but it is more difficult to explain the elevation of IgA. In order to settle the possible connection between the activity and immunopathogenesis of LGV and the elevation of IgA we are going to perform a longitudinal study in the acute cases of the present series, all of whom had received tetracycline treatment. In addition, a further study of the present patients with chronic LGV by the use of multiple immunological parameters will be performed.

SUMMARY

Fifty patients with lymphogranuloma venereum (LGV) were studied for the serum levels of the three immunoglobulins IgA, IgG and IgM. Ten of the patients were young men with an untreated LGV contracted within six months prior to the present examination, while the remaining forty patients had an old infection contracted twenty-four to forty-five years before the present study. Three of the latter forty patients still had an active LGV. By anamnestic and serologic evidence thirteen patients of the whole series were regarded to have had syphilis. IgA was found to be elevated in seven of the acute cases, in two of the old active cases and in ten of the presumably inactive cases. The corresponding figures for IgG were four, two and twelve, respectively. IgM was elevated in only four of the fifty cases: in two of the acute, in one of the old active and in one of the old inactive. In the presumably inactive cases the serum level of IgA and IgG seemed to be higher in the cases with a formerly more severe involvement of the intestine. Half of the cases of old inactive LGV with an elevated IgA had earlier had syphilis. It was suggested that an elevated IgA in patients with LGV might indicate an activity of the disease and the need for further treatment.

REFERENCES

Castenado, J. P. and Williams, R. C., Jr.: Anticomplementary activity of sera from patients with connective tissue disease and normal subjects. *J Lab Clin Med*, 69:217, 1967.

Delhanty, J. J. and Catterall, R. D.: Immunoglobulins in syphilis. *Lancet*, 2:1099, 1969.

Jersild, M.: Alterations des proteines seriques chez des malades atteints de lymphogranulomatose inguinale (Nicolas-Favre) et du syndrome genito-ano-rectal (Jersild). *Acta Derm Venereol*, 18:491, 1937.

Lassus, A.: Treponemal and lipoidal tests in old treated syphilis. *Acta Derm Venereol* (suppl), 48:60, 1968.

Lassus, A. and Mustakallio, K. K.: Anticomplementary activity in serological tests for syphilis as a clue to connective tissue diseases of an autoimmune nature. *Ann Clin Res*, 1:74, 1969.

Lassus, A., Mustakallio, K. K. and Wager, O.: Auto-immune serum factors and IgA elevation in lymphogranuloma venereum. *Ann Clin Res*, 2:51, 1970.

Laurell, A.-B., Oxelius, V.-A. and Rorsman, H.: Serum immunoglobulin levels in syphilis. *Acta Derm Venereol*, 48:268, 1968.

Mancini, G., Carbonara, A. O. and Heremans, J. F.: Immuno-chemical quantitation of antigens by single radial immuno-diffusion. *Immunochemistry*, 2:235, 1965.

Onisk, K.: Immunoglobulins in untreated early syphilis. *Br J Vener Dis*, 42:139, 1966.

Räsänen, J. A. and Wager, O.: A normal series for immunological aberrations. (Under preparation.)

Sheagren, J. N., Block, J. B., Trautman, J. R. and Wolff, S. M.: Immunologic reactivity in patients with leprosy. *Ann Intern Med*, 70:295, 1969.

Sonck, C. E.: Über die photosensibilität bei lymphogranuloma inguinale. *Acta Derm Venereol* (suppl), 22:6, 1941.

Tomasi, T. B., Jr. and Bienenstock, J.: Secretory immunoglobulins. *Adv Immunol*, 9:1, 1968.

Wager, O.: Immunological aspects of leprosy with special reference to autoimmune diseases. *Bull WHO*, 41:793, 1969.

Wager, O.: Unpublished observations.

Williams, R. D. and Gutman, A. B.: Hyperproteinemia with reversal of the albumin:globulin ratio in lymphogranuloma inguinale. *Proc Soc Exp Biol Med*, 34:91, 1936.

CHAPTER 14

ACCEPTANCE OF THE CONDOM AS A VENEREAL DISEASE PROPHYLACTIC

WILLIAM W. DARROW

INTRODUCTION TO THE PROBLEM

S EXUAL ABSTINENCE, in theory the most effective method of venereal disease prevention, has never been very popular in
practice. Charles II of England, allegedly the sire of no less than
twenty-nine illegitimate children, recognized that the highest
moral standards of sexual conduct were often very difficult to
uphold. In an effort to reduce the problems resulting from his
own wanton behavior, His Royal Highness instructed a physician
in his court to develop a device that would reduce the risks of
conception and venereal infection. The instrument invented by
Dr. Condom, which still bears his name, apparently was effective
to some degree, for its use eventually spread throughout the
world (Himes, 1963). Unfortunately for the sponsor of this
humanitarian adventure in applied research, the early models
were either defective or too late in coming to do him much
good.

After centuries of observation we in public health are beginning to realize, as Charles II recognized long before us, that
moral standards demanding sexual chastity outside of marriage
are often violated. When the United States entered World
War I, and large numbers of selectees drawn from all parts of
the country were examined, it was found that the venereal diseases constituted a leading cause for rejection (Vonderlehr and
Heller, 1946: 5-6). A more precise figure was placed on the vene-

real disease problem in World War II. As a result of a nation-wide selective service screening survey, one out of every twenty inductees was discovered to have a reactive blood test for syphilis (Vonderlehr and Usilton, 1942). Even more dramatic in terms of pointing out the discrepancy between avowed sexual standards and actual experiences were the widely read findings of Kinsey and his colleagues. Kinsey and others reported in 1948 that 73.1 percent of all American males by the age of twenty had engaged in premarital intercourse, at least 37 percent of the male population had some homosexual experience and about a third of the married men in all age groups admitted to extra-marital experiences. Faced with these figures, it was very difficult for us to continue to maintain that appeals for sexual continence were successfully preventing the acquisition and spread of the venereal diseases in American society (Cf. Hazen and others, 1940).

The Armed Forces of the United States have boldly led the search for viable alternatives to moral prophylaxis (Siler, 1943). As early as World War I, when the number of new cases of venereal disease in the Army exceeded by 100,000 the number of battlefield casualties (Parran and Vonderlehr, 1941), mechanical, chemical and chemical-therapeutic methods of prophylaxis were widely promoted. Where stringently employed, prophylactic measures were 99.7 percent effective in reducing the rates of venereal disease infection among American servicemen (Moore, 1943:560). However, there has been, until very recently, great resistance to adopting the proven military methods in civilian control efforts. The reasons for this reluctance appear to have been prudery and penicillin. Today, with pressing population problems and gonorrhea apparently out of control, the public seems to be more receptive to information about contraception and venereal disease prevention. With increasing evidence of antibiotic resistant organisms, Public Health officials seem to be more willing to accept comprehensive venereal disease control programs based on both treatment *and prevention*.

Concomitant with the liberalization of sexual attitudes in American society (Reiss, 1970), we have recently conducted a study of health behavior patterns which focused on the actions people take to prevent themselves from acquiring a venereal disease. In the broadest sense, our study has attempted to answer the question, "Can venereal disease be prevented?" In a narrower sense, we asked three related questions: (a) How many people are now using the condom? (b) How many people will accept the rubber sheath when it is defined (or redefined) to them as a venereal disease prophylactic? and (c) How many cases of venereal disease will be prevented among those people who accept, and report regular use of, the prophylactic?

GENERAL HYPOTHESES

Since our review of the literature revealed that the use-effectiveness of the condom as a venereal disease prophylactic had never been adequately evaluated in a field trial, we entered this investigation with very few assumptions. Available data showed that the incidence of infectious venereal disease in the United States had increased considerably during the period 1957 to 1970. Figure XIV-1 shows, on a logarithmic scale, the rates of change for reported cases of gonorrhea and infectious syphilis. Gonorrhea steadily increased from 214,872 reported cases in 1957 to 600,072 reported cases in calendar year 1970. Primary and secondary syphilis increased from 6,581 cases in 1957 to 21,982 reported cases in calendar year 1970. The syphilis eradication effort mounted in the early sixties apparently served to slow down the rate of increase in the middle of the decade, but early syphilis cases are rising once again. Male and female trends changed consistently.

Available data also showed trends in contraceptive use among American women in the eighteen to thirty-nine year old age range over this same period of time. Table 14-I shows percentage distributions for the various contraceptive methods available to the American market before and after the introduction of the *Pill* and the intrauterine device (I.U.D.) In 1955, 39 percent of the women surveyed reported use of the condom or a foam, jelly or douche, all of which may have had some prophylactic value against sexually-transmitted diseases. Oral contraceptive agents were introduced for consumption in 1960 and intrauterine devices became available in 1964. By 1965, 26 percent of the women still

Cases of Infectious Venereal Disease Reported By Sex: 1957–1970

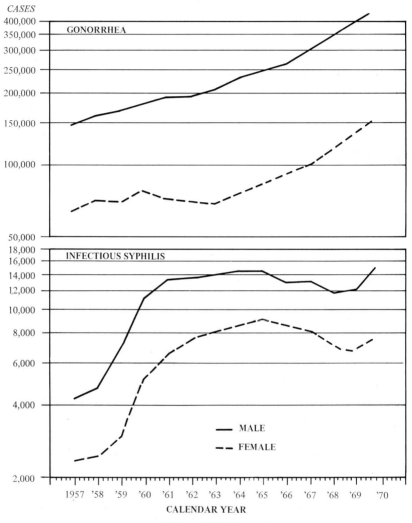

Figure XIV-1

TABLE 14-I

TRENDS IN CONTRACEPTIVE USE AMONG SELECTED SAMPLES
OF AMERICAN WOMEN, 1955-1971

	National Samples			VD Clinic Patients
Methods Now Using	1955[1] (percent)	1965[1] (percent)	1970[2] (percent)	1971[3] (percent)
Oral contraceptive	—	24	64.5	47.5
I.U.D. (coil, loop, etc.)	—	1	8.9	10.5
Diaphragm	25	10	6.7	2.5
Douche, foam, jelly	12	8	5.5	5.3
Condom	27	18	3.1	2.6
Rhythm-withdrawal	29	18	3.9	2.6
Sterilization	2	5	4.8	0.0
No method	—	—	2.7	18.4
Multiple or unknown	5	16	—	10.5
	100	100	100.0	100.0
	N = 1,901	N = 2,445	N = 3,240 (Physicians)	N = 38

SOURCES:
1. Westoff, C. F. and Ryder, N. B., "United States: Methods of Fertility Control, 1955, 1960, and 1965." *Studies in Family Planning* 17 (February, 1967):3.
2. "A.A.M.C.H. Survey Results: 97% of Obstetricians and Gynecologists Favor Use of Oral Contraceptive." A.A.M.C.H. Newsletter (May, 1970):3.
3. Sacramento Special Study, Pretest Results.

had some protection against venereal disease, but by 1970, only 9.6 percent had a modicum of protection. This evidence strongly suggests an association between the changing patterns of contraceptive use and the growing problem of infectious venereal disease in the United States.

We expected that an even smaller proportion of the patients seen in a venereal disease clinic would be using the condom, foam, jelly, or douche. In a small sample of thirty-eight women, we found only three patients who were currently using these products for contraceptive purposes. The lone female who always insisted that her sex partners use a condom, had no children, no history of venereal disease and had come to clinic as an *extra precaution*. She was found to have no evidence of disease. The data shown in the last column are taken from the pretest of our study and are only suggestive, but we predict that the final results of the survey will support the hypothesis that the condom, jelly, cream, and douche offer significant protection against the venereal diseases while the Pill and I.U.D. offer no protection at all.

ACCEPTANCE OF THE CONDOM

Assuming that the use-effectiveness of the condom can be demonstrated, the problem of motivating sexually active adults to protect themselves against the venereal diseases by using the rubber sheath remains. The objections to condom use may seem too difficult to overcome, yet there is in the literature some cause for optimism.

None of the deleterious side effects associated with the Pill (nausea, irregular bleeding and weight gain) are found with the condom. This fact alone probably accounts for the lower drop out rate among married couples adopting the condom as a contraceptive (27 percent over a three year period) (Tietze and Gamble, 1944) as opposed to the Pill (34 percent over a two year period) (Corkey, 1964). Also, the contraceptive rate of change per 100 years of use has been shown to be lower for the condom (6.7) than any of the other "traditional" methods (Westoff and others, 1961). Hence, once a couple adopts the condom as their contraceptive of choice, they tend to stick with it.

Secondly, the condom is the only recognized, highly reliable contraceptive which does not require a prescription to buy. Since it can be purchased from a vending machine in many areas, the condom can often be obtained without any embarrassing social interaction taking place (Calderone, 1962).

Thirdly, the condom seems particularly well suited to people who are classified as lower class and who tend to visit public clinics. In terms of temporal sequence, the condom is directly associated with the sexual act while the once-a-day Pill often is not. Rainwater (1960:58) has noted, "The most widely accepted method, the condom, is also the one that is most easily understood, the one that seems the least mysterious and magical." Since many of the people studied by Rainwater believed that the man planted the fertile egg during intercourse, he argued that the rubber sheath which captured the "egg" left most couples assured that a pregnancy would not result. More importantly, Rainwater (1965) observed in a later study that lower class families tend to form segregated role sets in which the man is held responsible for initiating sexual activity and providing protection. Shimoni (1968) has argued that family planning programs have largely overlooked the role played by men in the sexual act. Recent research has shown that men designated as underprivileged want to share the burden in fertility control (Arnold and Cogswell, 1970) and are quite willing to cooperate in fertility control efforts (Kangas, 1969).

Table II shows condom acceptance rates for the 101 Public Health Clinic patients who completed a questionnaire during the week of pretest. Although the pretest schedules were six or seven pages long, and took about twenty minutes to complete, only ten (9 percent of the patients) failed to return the questionnaires. The offer of three lubricated and three regular condoms was made to all subjects, regardless of sex, diagnosis or willingness to cooperate in the study. As seen in Table 14-II, thirty-six males (57 percent of the total) and fifteen females (39 percent of the total) accepted the offer.

Of the 101 patients who came to the clinic specifically for a

TABLE 14-II

CONDOM ACCEPTANCE AMONG VD CLINIC PATIENTS BY
METHODS OF CONTRACEPTION AND SEX, SACRAMENTO
SPECIAL STUDY, PRETEST RESULTS

Methods Used	*Male*		*Female*		*Totals*
	Acceptance	*Rejection*	*Acceptance*	*Rejection*	
Oral contraceptive	10	5	7	10	32
I.U.D. (coil, loop)	0	0	2	2	4
Diaphragm	0	1	0	0	1
Douche, foam, jelly	1	0	0	1	2
Rhythm-withdrawal	4	1	1	1	7
Multiple methods	4	0	2	0	6
Other*	0	1	1	0	2
Nothing	8	4	2	5	19
Unknown	9	15	0	4	28
	36	27	15	23	101

* Vasectomy and Condom

venereal disease check-up, thirty-five males and twenty-nine females (63 percent of the pretest sample) reported that they or their sex partners *never* used a prophylactic. One young man reported that he never used condoms because, in his own words, "they're a hassle to buy." Another wrote that he occasionally used rubbers, but only as a joke, and apparently tiring of the jest, rejected the free sample. Although we were very careful to point out the potential prophylactic value of condom use, one very lovely Lolita-like lass, perhaps recalling her recent visits to the family dentist, innocently purred as she seductively slipped the two packs of threes in a waist pocket, "I'd rather have a lollipop."

I don't believe that the prophylactic value of lollipops has ever been demonstrated, but you will see in Table II that more than half of the patients relying on the Pill for contraceptive purposes accepted a complimentary supply of prophylactics. All six of the patients using multiple methods accepted and five out of seven relying on rhythm or withdrawal picked up the packages we offered. The only category showing total rejection was represented by a male who reported that his usual sex partner used a diaphragm.

The patients were provided with the prophylactics before the laboratory evidence became available to confirm the clinical diagnosis. It was found that 32 of the 101 patients were infected with gonorrhea and not one showed evidence of an untreated syphilis infection. We expected that gonorrhea patients would be more likely to accept the products than their noninfected peers. No differences were discovered. Half of the gonorrhea patients and half of the noninfected patients accepted.

SUMMARY AND CONCLUSIONS

In closing, let me point out once again that these findings are tentative. In the final analysis, we shall thoroughly examine all the data collected from 2,190 VD clinic patients, 175 Neighborhood Health Center visitors and 708 community residents in order to understand health behavior practices, particularly as they relate to venereal disease prevention. Preliminary findings have been cited to suggest that people in high risk of acquiring a venereal disease rarely take adequate precautions, but that many, when offered the opportunity, are quite willing to initiate preventive care. On the other hand, a condom distribution program certainly cannot be considered to be the final solution to the venereal disease problem. The rubber sheath may turn out to be effective in preventing cases of venereal disease, but our preliminary findings clearly show that the condom is not everyone's bag.

REFERENCES

Arnold, C. B. and Cogswell, B. E.: A condom distribution program for adolescents. *Am J Public Health,* 61:739-750, 1971.

Calderone, M. S.: An inventory of contraceptive methods adapted to public health practice. *Am J Public Health,* 52:1712-1719, 1962.

Corkey, E. C.: A family planning program for the low-income family. *J Marriage and the Family,* 26:478-480, 1964.

Hazen, H. H., *et al.*: The chemical and mechanical prevention of syphilis and gonorrhea. *J Vener Dis Inform,* 21:311-313, 1940.

Himes, N. E.: *Medical History of Contraception.* New York, Gamut Pr, 1963.

Kangas, L. W.: *A Condom Distribution Program to Reduce Unwanted Teenage Pregnancies.* Chapel Hill, North Carolina School of Public Health, 1969.

Kinsey, A. C., Pomeroy, W. B. and Martin, C. E.: *Sexual Behavior in the Human Male.* Philadelphia, Saunders, 1948.

Moore, J. E.: *The Modern Treatment of Syphilis,* 2nd ed. Springfield, Thomas, 1943.

Parran, T. and Vonderlehr, R. A.: *Plain Words About Venereal Disease.* New York, Reynal and Hitchcock, 1941.

Rainwater, L.: *And the Poor Get Children.* Chicago, Quadrangle, 1960.

Rainwater, L.: *Family Design: Marital Sexuality, Family Size and Contraception.* Chicago, Aldine, 1965.

Reiss, I. L.: How and why America's sex standards are changing. In Gagnon, John H. and Simon, William (eds.): *The Sexual Scene.* Chicago, Aldine, 1970, p. 43-57.

Shimoni, K.: *Selected Correlates of Condom Use Among Urban Negro Males.* Mimeographed, Chapel Hill, North Carolina Department of Maternal and Child Health, School of Public Health, 1968.

Siler, J. F.: The prevention and control of venereal diseases in the Army of the United States of America. *Army Med Bull,* 67: entire issue, 1943.

Tietze, C. and Gamble, C. J.: The condom as a contraceptive method in public health work. *Hum Fertility,* 9:97-111, 1944.

Vonderlehr, R. A. and Heller, J. R., Jr.: *The Control of Venereal Disease.* New York, Reynal and Hitchcock, 1946.

Vonderlehr, R. A. and Usilton, L. J.: Syphilis among men of draft age in the United States. *JAMA,* 120:1369-1372, 1942.

AUTHOR INDEX

227

SUBJECT INDEX